QUESTIONS & ANSWERS

Questions & Answers

Explaining the Basic Principles and Standards of
THE BACH FLOWER REMEDIES®

John Ramsell

Trustee and Curator of
The Dr Edward Bach Centre & Healing Trust

SAFFRON WALDEN
THE C. W. DANIEL COMPANY LIMITED

First published in Great Britain by
The Dr Edward Bach Centre
1986
This completely revised edition was
published by
The C. W. Daniel Company Limited
1 Church Path, Saffron Walden,
Essex, England
1991

ISBN 0 85207 240 6

Designed and Produced in association with
Book Production Consultants, Cambridge, England
Typeset by Rowland Phototypesetting Limited
Bury St Edmunds, Suffolk
Printed in England by
St Edmundsbury Press Limited,
Bury St Edmunds, Suffolk

This book has been produced on
part re-cycled paper

CONTENTS

TO WHOM IT MAY CONCERN

We would like to state categorically that the Bach Remedies are prepared from non-poisonous wild flowers – they are benign in their action, and can be taken by people of all ages with absolute impunity.

The purpose of these flowers is to establish an equilibrium between one's higher self, mind and body, so that when emotional upsets retard general progress, the correcting of the emotional states in a gentle way by means of specifically related flowers allow the person to progress accordingly, thus acting as an adjunct to treatment that might already have been prescribed by a physician. These Flower Remedies do not take the place of orthodox medicine and if any relativity between a physical condition and form of outlook is referred to in books written on the subject, such mention is intended to reflect only in keeping with the above explanation – no claim is made to actually treat or cure physical ailments as such.

We always advise that clients see their medical doctors. The Bach Remedies are not advertised nor do we solicit in any form – clients approach us and in turn we advise fully our position so that no false impression or misleading advice is offered. It might be added that the Bach Remedies have been in being for over 50 years and their successful efficacious application throughout the world would be vouched for by thousands of professional as well as lay people.

The Bach Flower Remedies® The Bach Centre

MOUNT VERNON, a little house and garden, unpretentious in its appearance, yet known to thousands throughout the world as 'The Bach Centre', set in a picturesque village nestling in the Thames Valley, 10 miles south of Oxford, where Dr. Bach, Physician, Homoeopath, Harley Street Specialist and Consultant Bacteriologist finally lived and worked, perfecting his life's work of discovery 38 non-poisonous wild flowers. Each of the 38 remedies is correlated to a specific negative state of mind, personality trait, mood or temperament, that so often prove to be the real cause, psychosomatically, in the break down of one's physical and mental equilibrium.

The original team of helpers who worked with Dr. Bach were Nora Weeks and Victor Bullen – both absolutely dedicated to the work and discoveries of their beloved mentor. Nora was herself a professional radiographer, often finding herself working under Dr. Bach during an appointment at one of the London hospitals. She was so taken with the man's sincere outlook and great sensitivity of purpose and genuine concern for his patients that she wasn't at all surprised to find herself 'leaving' her professional work at the doctor's invitation, to accompany him in his great quest when he too gave up his lucrative Harley Street practice, in search of the natural healing qualities he was destined to find, embodied in the heart of Nature itself.

Nora witnessed the whole spectrum of Dr. Bach's discoveries first hand – proving herself to be not only his right hand helper, but someone he could rely on to nurture him during the great development of his increasing sensitivity through the latter 4 years of his life. Her dedication and loving respect for the doctor must be recorded as perhaps the back-bone of his endeavour, for without her supportive resilience it can safely be assumed that the doctor's work might have faltered before completion – for he did indeed suffer greatly, both mentally and physically as an integral part of his great discovery. The doctor bequeathed to her the whole responsibility of his work, saying to her at one stage, "I have nearly completed my work and I won't be with you much longer". And so, when the final Remedy had been found, he passed on, asking Nora to ensure that the 38 Remedies remain intact in their own entity because he proclaimed them to be complete, covering every negative state of mind known to man.

For over 40 years Nora, with the help of Victor (a dear soul, a reservoir of laughter, music and love) continued steadfastly to offer the Bach Remedies to the world – never succumbing to the many persuasive ideas that cropped up from time to time, keeping the work pure and ever simple as intended by the doctor, protecting the principle and methodology from many who would wish to redetermine the concept in some vision of their own making.

Nora passed on in 1978 after Victor had preceded her a couple of years earlier. They brought into partnership the present curators who now carry the full responsibility of the work in the same vein and spirit of dedication.

No advertising has been introduced even during these latter years, but the increased interest in the Bach therapy has grown, by word of mouth alone, to such great proportion that distributors had to be established in different countries to help cope with the demand. The old system of despatching the little packages to all and sundry, in answer to individual orders, is (except for the U.K.) a thing of the past – but nevertheless, the Centre is still available to those who require further information or help, for the basic preparation of each of the mother tinctures from the original flower locations discovered by Dr. Bach is still carried out there. The authoritative knowledge remains within the Centre, and visitors are seen by appointment, to have a little chat and a further enlightenment (if required) about the whole aspect of Dr. Bach's life and work, as well as to see the furniture that the doctor made by hand, and to 'feel' the atmosphere of the little consulting room that has always been used for this purpose.

The Bach Centre – Mount Vernon, can be summed up as the OAK TREE that stands firm and will ever remain the strength of a great man's gift to the world. Twigs have, over the years, been broken off in the hope of producing facsimiles, but to no avail because the origin of Dr. Bach is far too firmly established, with roots embedded in the suffering, both mental and physical, endured by him in bringing to fruition the very purpose of his existence on earth.

Postscript:
Although a lot has happened over the years, one wonders, if in fact, events ever really do change, because nothing has altered in relation to the Bach Centre, in its appearance, its furnishings or indeed its activities.

We are fully dedicated to this very day to the principles of Dr. Bach in that we make no charge for our time in any way – consultations (most extend to one or two hours) are free, even the cost of the treatment bottle is waived for the elderly or those of poor circumstances – inability to pay is of no consequence at all. Our day seminars are gratuitiously offered (including teas and biscuits). We have been granted the registration of a Charitable Trust which will also take into its keeping, the old non-charitable trust that is Mount Vernon – this will ensure that the little house and garden will for all time (as was originally intended), remain as the established Centre and original home of Dr. Bach's work. We aim to support the Charity from our own funds and through its benevolence, perhaps partly reciprocate the accrued benefits that the ever increasing demand for Dr Bach's findings have created.

THE BACH FLOWER REMEDIES – a simple and natural method of establishing equilibrium and harmony through the personality by means of non-poisonous wild flowers, discovered by: Edward Bach, MB, BS, MRCS., LRCP., DP.

The Bach Remedies – established in 1936 – act as a form of supportive therapy, and having proved themselves in this form for an unblemished 50 years or more (not a word of complaint ever of any consequence), they are now in great demand throughout the world as a non-medicinal adjunct to various forms of treaments (including Allopathy). They are therefore an integral part of the whole healing spectrum, not as an alternative or interfering vehicle, but as a very respected complement to many restorative treatments and therapies. We are often called upon by doctors (GP's included), Veterinarians, Dentists, manipulative specialists, psyco-therapists and so on, to supply the Remedies either for use within their own particular service, or direct to their clients for whom the bach Flower Remedies, in their opinion, would prove to be beneficial. We provide this service unsolicited – therapists learn the value of the Remedies mainly through favourable word-of-mouth recommendation, and so in turn, send to us for further details, and after initial trials find that the Remedies work in their own quiet way, as a harmless, non-addictive, non-side effect support to a particular aspect of their treatment that normally would not be considered in their standard diagnosis, e.g. subservience, hatred, envy, jealousy, self recrimination, guilt, arrogance, intolerance, impatience, procrastination, as well as rigidity of attitude and mind, autocratic outlook and behaviour, pride, apathy, embitterment with one's lot in life ('poor old me') and so on. They are benign in their action and result in no unpleasant reactions. They can be taken by persons of all ages, and have proved to be very effective for animals and plant life.

Genuine Bach Flower Remedies will be recognizable by the use of Dr. Bach's original signature *"Bach"* in the working title. Please beware of dilutions, facsimiles and replicas that purport to be *'equal to'* or *'the same as'* or that claim to hold some contemporary association to Dr. Bach's discoveries and method of preparation – such products are **not Bach Flower Remedies**.

General Information

Do you run Seminars or Courses?

In the past, the Centre felt it was unnecessary to conduct courses on the subject simply because the books were self explanatory and if further advice be sought, we at the Bach Centre were only too happy to expound our knowledge accordingly.

With the ever growing interest and demand for the Remedies, with people thirsting for more and deeper insight into the history of the work, we have now commenced to offer seminars in the form of 'A day out at the Bach Centre' when visitors have the opportunity to visit Dr. Bach's little home, Mount Vernon, see his hand-made furniture and some of his original Mother Tincture preparations and writings, as well as enjoy slides, video and general dicussion in keeping with the subject. This has become possible through the transference of the production aspect of the work to a separate 'production unit' nearby – the old production room having been converted into an ideal seminar room.

With more time to devote to the finer side of the work, we are also able to introduce short courses at the Centre. The reason for what might appear to be a 'U-turn' in policy is simply that we need to be able to recommend alternative addresses to those who would prefer to obtain direct and personal attention within a reasonable travelling distance – not everyone can journey to Mount Vernon. In providing a general enlightenment on the subject, with the emphasis on using the correct methods of prescribing as laid down by Dr. Bach, we would then be happy to make a recommendation knowing at least that the practitioner would conform to the purity and original methodology when prescribing the remedies.

General information on seminars and courses can be obtained from the Centre (Details of courses/seminars abroad can be obtained from our respective distributors, listed on page 117).

Which books do you recommend I read to begin with?

There are a number of books available on the subject of the Bach Remedies which generally are self-explanatory and allow most people to avail themselves of this particular therapy without having to seek out the aid of a 'specialist'. It was Dr. Bach's intention that the explanation of his work be put in such simple terms that anyone, no matter their station in life, would be able to understand and use the Remedies without fear of them being beyond their comprehension. Nevertheless – our experience tells us that there are some who would still wish to gain a further knowledge in relation to the wider spectrum of each of the Bach Remedies, so let this little booklet act as an informative guide in helping to establish a firmer understanding by fitting the stray pieces of the jig-saw in their rightful place and thereby allowing the reticent to take the first step with confidence.

Here each book is described briefly:

1. **"Twelve Healers"**. This booklet is *the* essential booklet – it is the 'Bible' as far as the Bach Remedies are concerned, for it offers Dr. Bach's own description of each remedy, and any other written in this vein is, by comparison, but a complementary adjunct to the doctor's offering.

2. **"Heal Thyself"**. Written by Dr. Bach – reflecting his profound and beautiful philosophy, and intentionally

worded so as to ensure that its wonderful message is easily understood by all.

3. **"B.F.R. Step by Step"**. A complete guide to prescribing by Judy Howard. Step by Step is a comprehensive guide to the Bach Flower system. It is ideal for beginners who are new to the therapy, but also offers a wealth of additional insight for those already familiar with the subject.

4. **"Questions and Answers"**. This booklet by John Ramsell, answers questions one might have on the Remedies. It deals with general matters, prescribing and the use of the Remedies, alcoholics/drug addicts, pregnancy and little children, general data and standard policy and correct use of the Bach Remedies. Many years of experience have gone into this compilation.

Note: The above four booklets represent a cross-section of information that we consider to be important to the beginner'.

5. **"The Bach Remedies Repertory"**. You do not prescribe from this booklet, it is purely meant as a form of index when one is 'not quite certain' of one's proper choice. In this booklet the various states of mind are listed *first* with a recommendation of remedies that might apply. You then check each of the suggested remedies in one of the prescribing books (e.g. "Twelve Healers", "Step by Step", "The Handbook") to see which one if any is applicable. This is quite a helpful aid but it must be accepted that the picture offered is not necessarily complete.

6. **"Dictionary of the Bach Flower Remedies"**. Another booklet intended to aid the novice, in that it depicts the negative and positive aspects of each remedy in turn. The

object is simply this – if you are in the negative column you might require the remedy, if in the positive – you don't.

7. "**Handbook of the B.F.R. Illustrated**". This book is another that deals with prescribing, but describes the Remedies in depth, with case histories added for information. Also included in this book is a complete range of the Bach Flowers in the form of coloured illustrations, painted, many years ago, by Nora Harrison from the actual plants. The book was compiled by Dr. P. M. Chancellor, the content being a compilation of Nora Weeks' descriptions and case histories as printed over the years in the Bach News Letters – Dr. Chancellor thought it a good idea to combine this very helpful information under the one cover, and Nora Weeks happily granted him permission.

8. "**Medical Discoveries of Edward Bach, Physician**". Nora Weeks' biography of Dr. Bach. Only she could have written it, for she worked with the doctor in his professional days and accompanied him in his quest, witnessing the whole discovery first hand and being entrusted with the continuation of the work after the doctor's passing in 1936.

9. "**The Benefits of the B.F.R.**". Written by a long established and good friend of Nora Weeks. Her little booklet is not for prescribing, but it is a lovely enlightenment of what the work represents.

10. "**The Bach Remedy News Letter**". This is a regular 'letter' containing points of interest including news, announcements, case histories, developments from home and abroad. It is our means of keeping in touch with everyone – and there are three issues per annum – April, August and December.

11. **"Story of Mount Vernon"**. A booklet by Judy Howard, that conveys to the reader a history of this little house and especially the dedication of Dr. Bach's original team – Nora Weeks and Victor Bullen during their 40 odd years at Mount Vernon. They deserve recognition of their respective roles in the continuation and development of Dr. Bach's work, for without them the Bach Remedies would not have survived.

12. **"The Bach Flower Remedies. Illustrations and Preparations"** by Nora Weeks and Victor Bullen (friends and colleagues of Dr. Edward Bach). Nora Weeks and Victor Bullen worked with Dr. Bach and it was to them that the responsibility of his work was bequeathed. In 1964, as a tribute to the doctor's work, they published this book to share with others the essence of Nature within the Bach Flower Remedies. This new edition, with coloured photographs, was published in 1990.

13. **"The Original Writings of Edward Bach"**. Compiled from the Archives of the Dr. Edward Bach Healing Trust. This book, compiled by the curators and trustees of the Dr. Edward Bach Healing Trust, offers a most enlightening and intimate appreciation of this great physician. All the documents reproduced in this book are from the originals held by the Healing Trust at the Dr. Edward Bach Centre.

14. A Poster Chart of the Bach Flower Remedies (17½" x 25") is available in full colour. It explains the positive and negative aspects of the Remedies in the form of a large circular wheel, with illustrations of each flower at the periphary of each segment of the circle.

(Foreign editions of our literature are listed on page 119).

How long do the remedies keep?

If not used – the stock concentrates will keep indefinitely providing they are not abused in any way. Storage can be in a cupboard, situated in a cool place. Should a sediment form over a period of time, it is quite harmless and can be filtered off if one feels the need to do so. It might be of interest that we still have a range of Dr. Bach's original mother tinctures at the Centre – and they are as potent today as they were those many years ago. (No responsibility can be accepted for any deterioration of the brandy preservative)

Can the Remedies help in Dentistry?

Yes indeed. We are finding a growing interest in the Remedies these days, shown by dentists. Rescue Remedy is a good basic remedy to take prior to the event if there is some panic and trepidation. If very apprehensive and anxious, then Aspen will help too, and if the thought goes round and round in one's head like a long playing record, this can be relieved by including White Chestnut. One checks one's feelings and attitude and chooses the remedies accordingly. Carry some of the mixture with you to sip whilst at the dentist and if the dentist doesn't mind, (you are, it must be remembered, *his* patient), 4 drops of RR direct from your stock bottle to the glass of mouth wash will help to enhance your natural recuperative powers.

What are the 'Seven Bach Nosodes' – and do you supply them?

(Note: A Nosode is a Homoeopathic term loosely meaning antidote).

When Dr. Bach was still a Harley Street specialist, he also worked for some time in the laboratories of the Royal Homoeopathic Hospital and whilst there became interested in the relationship between intestinal toxaemia and chronic disease. He then isolated seven groups of intestinal flora and prepared nosodes from them homoeopathically, giving them to his patients by mouth. Their purpose was to cleanse and purify the intestinal tract and they proved to be most successful. However, during the course of his practical use of the nosodes, Dr. Bach noticed that he gave certain nosodes to certain types of people and that his patients formed seven distinct groups to which one of the seven nosodes applied. The seven groups were named by Dr. Bach and those same titles became the seven headings in his booklet "The Twelve Healers" because they all related to the various forms of outlook, temperament, type, personality etc. that were to be the basis of his further work and subsequent discoveries. The Bach Nosodes (known also as the 'Seven Bowel Nosodes') are still used today by some Homoeopathic hospitals and doctors throughout the world – but we at Mount Vernon do not handle them because they are akin to physical disease.

With the advent of so many new diseases today, would Bach, had he been alive, discovered more remedies?

The answer is that as the Remedies are not associated with physical states as such, new diseases would hold no significance. We emphasize in all our literature that the Bach Flower Remedies relate to the outlook, personality, temperament of a person – see for example explanation on pages 50 to 53. The Introduction to this booklet also states that Dr. Bach decreed his work to be complete (also see bottom of page 56), a fact that has been borne out ever since.

Rumour has it that some plants are no longer available – Elm for instance due to the Dutch Elm disease – Is this true?

The Elm, now growing again in this area but not yet flowering, is still flourishing in other areas – it means our having to travel, but that is of no consequence. Other 'elusive' plants have demanded a prolonged search before new growths have come to light, a test no doubt of our fortitude and patience, but we have never yet been let down – Faith has always seen us through.

Are the Bach Remedies classed as an alternative or a complementary therapy?

If one had to choose, they would certainly be complementary simply because they can be taken alongside or work as an adjunct to other forms of treatment, be it Homoeopathic or Allopathic. (Therein lies one answer to the next question).

Will the Bach Remedies interfere with other forms of medicinal treatment.

No . . . because they work on the mental/spiritual level and will not interfere with the curing of the body by other measures – they in fact hasten recovery by tackling the psychogenic aspect of a person's illness, which relates to the real cause!

How did Dr. Bach discover the flowers – was it scientific, experimental or what?

There was obviously the necessity for research and some experimentation (on himself) in the early days – his Homoeopathic knowledge of plants, his study of Nature and essentially his great sensitivity and intuition set him on the road to discovering his first 19 Remedies. Later, during his latter 2 years, after he had settled at Mount Vernon, he discovered his final 19 Remedies – only, during this period, he began also to suffer states of mental anguish (extreme in some cases) and a subsequent physical discomfort (created by mental pressures) before finding the antidotal Remedy.

Dr. Bach was in the same mould as Pasteur and Hahnemann, who courageously pioneered themselves to find the cure to some disease or illness. There was, in Dr. Bach's case, one subtle difference perhaps, in that conditions of mind cannot, as in the case of poisons or germs, be self inflicted – so the inducement had to come from some 'other source' and that could only mean from a 'Higher level'. Once having been given the condition, he was then *led* to find the cure.

How do the Remedies work?

Such a question has been answered many times in different ways depending on the particular avenue of interest or vocation of the enquirer. We think that most aware people are convinced that life is composed of a Oneness – a unity of Higher-self, mind and body, and in obtaining a balance or equilibrium embracing all three, then the body (created as the most perfect healing machine) would be allowed to do its job properly. It is when there is disharmony that the door opens to allow disease, weakness, depression and so on to enter. The purpose of the Remedies is to bring back that natural even keel once more, so that a being can progress in all aspects of one's destiny. Some souls nevertheless would find that their true awareness might not have developed as far as others – this cannot be forced, because progress in this is dependent on one's level of evolution. We have all reached our own status of spiritual development and cannot go further until our present lessons and experiences have been mastered (the very object of our present incarnation).

One can think of no better reply than that given by Dr. Bach during a lecture at Southport in 1934. He said: "The action of these Remedies is to raise our vibrations and open up our channels for the reception of our Spiritual Self; to flood our natures with the particular virtue we need, and wash out from us the fault which is causing harm. They are able, like beautiful music or any glorious uplifting thing which gives us inspiration, to raise our very natures, and bring us nearer to our souls, and by that very act bring us peace and relieve our sufferings. They cure, not by attacking disease, but by flooding our bodies with the beautiful vibrations of our Higher Nature, in the presence of whom disease melts away as snow in the sunshine."

Some say the Remedies have a placebo effect – is that true?

No – this can be disproved in the successful use of the remedies on animals and little children. Often too, people in an extremely irritable mood, or vile temper are helped successfully – and they certainly would not be receptive to any form of auto-suggestion.

Are they habit forming, do they have side effects?

The answer is 'NO' in both cases. They can be taken by people of all ages and there is no danger of an overdose or side effects. Even should the wrong choice be made, no harm would ensue. (See also question on reactions – page 59).

What is the correct pronunciation of the doctor's name – as the composer or as 'Batch'?

Many people still ask this question, especially our Welsh friends who say, quite rightly, it should be pronounced in the guttural – in the 'Welsh way', where it means 'little' or 'dear' – for the doctor's family originally came from

29

Wales many years ago. When Dr. Bach began his medical training at University College Hospital, his fellow students, mostly English, and therefore unable to pronounce his name correctly, decided on 'Batch', and by this name he has been called, ever since. We at Mount Vernon obviously continue in the same vein as we have been 'brought up' in that way – but we do nevertheless accept both pronunciations, for not everyone would be expected to know the little story behind the name.

Are the Remedies adversely affected by pollution, also do X-Ray machines at airports cause any deterioration?

Nearly all the flowers and trees are within easy striking distance of Mount Vernon – most of them in very close proximity. The Centre is in the heart of beautiful rural countryside and so pollution in a heavy sense does not interfere with the surrounding wild plants . . . nevertheless, there indeed must be crop spraying – maybe acid rain and so on to contend with, although we do our utmost to stay clear of it all where we can. Having said that – it must also be remembered that the flowers are *not ingested* in any way, it is the Life Force of the plant that is extracted, a healing that is omni-potent, the ultimate power itself, the quality of which cannot be increased or decreased by man's interfering methods. We can liken it to ourselves when we abuse our bodies by taking drugs, alcohol or general over-indulgence – even to the extreme result of shortening our own lives, yet, despite all this harm to our physical beings, *our* Life Force, Soul or whatever, will continue irrespective – unharmed! Similarly with plants – the Life Force will remain unscathed and pure despite man's irresponsible and careless actions.

The healing quality of the flowers, as explained in the preceding paragraph has a great bearing on the efficacy of the remedies remaining, even when subjected to X-ray clearance. Obviously if one has the choice to have them hand-inspected rather than have them put through the machine then do so, but the remedies have been going to different countries throughout the world for nearly 55 years, suffering the various routine tests and checks that are periodically required. There has never been any suggestion of loss of efficacy at any time which affirms the fact that the vibrational healing level remains intact.

How much do I charge? (Many prescribers ask this question because they feel there is a need to comform to Bach's standards)

We sometimes learn of good people helping others with the Remedies and making no charge whatsoever for their offering, despite the fact that it can be a strain on their personal resources. Dr. Bach's great benevolence and compassion is of course known to all who have made a study of his life, and some dear souls feel they should image themselves in that same mould when it comes to payment for services rendered. Dr. Bach at the beginning, held little clinics in a hired hall and treated people without charge, but as time progressed he realized that the reason few people attended his gathering was due to their suspicion of being offered 'something for nothing'. So – he then decided to leave a plate for his patients to donate something if they so wished, but even this experiment fell flat and all he ended up with were a few odd coins and a lovely selection of buttons! From then on he charged a nominal fee for his remedies and so people began to come to him, for his work had now taken on an air of 'respectability' – but at least they would still gain the benefit of treatment, this being his only concern. Mind you – it goes without saying, that he still gave away his treatment whenever the least excuse offered itself, most especially to the aged and poor.

So, those of you concerned, please don't worry about having to charge something, if only to cover expenses.

Many visitors to the Centre hope that they can choose a day when the Remedies are being made.

Unfortunately this is not so easy as it sounds. The most important factor is of course the perfect state of the plant, but this must culminate with ideal weather conditions. This means that our actual preparations are often carried out on a spot decision – we simply pack up our gear and ride off into the countryside somewhere, having dropped everything to do this. It is impossible for us to forecast in advance any particular day when we might attempt to make a remedy – our weather is far too inclement for that, and time is so precious to us these days that our opportunities have to be taken as they arise which rather excludes planning for the benefit of interested observers. (Also see reference on page 118).

What is the significance of the figures 1–20 and 1–40 on some of your labels?

These references indicate the ratio of the basic flower to water content in the original make up of the Mother Tincture preparations – one related to the Sun Method and the other to the Boiling Method. They are pharmaceutical terms required by law, but hold no actual bearing to the taking of the remedies or the content of the prepared stock bottles – so please don't concern yourself in any way. For directions, follow the instructions on our printed form or (if stated), on the label.

I understand that you have different labels for different countries, is that correct?

As you will appreciate – various countries have different laws governing the import and distribution of the Bach Remedies. We have to conform to their requirements and so labels have to be made up accordingly. The UK label states 'purchased in the UK' – this is to safeguard some inadvertent infringement of 'unathorised' foriegn distribution by anyone in Great Britain. Our overseas distributors have worked extremely hard to establish in their respective countries the acceptance of the Bach Remedies officially, that is why we need to strictly adhere to the rules of exporting that their hard earned licences allow.

We understand that you have established a production unit which is run under separate management – does this alter the quality of the Remedies in any way?

Due to lack of space, we at Mount Vernon had reached the stage where we were no longer capable of carrying the weight of production equal to the demand, in addition to all the other responsibilities that it was our duty as curators and trustees to perform. So it became necessary for us to shed the bonds of the 'business aspect' that was threatening to consume most of our precious time, a development we could not accept, and so changes had to be made.

Dr. Bach was personally acquainted with the family of A. Nelson, the renowned Homoeopathic Company, and chose to use their facilities for the purpose of bottling and sale of the prepared stock remedies. To this end he would send them as and when required, supplies of his Mother Tinctures. Nelsons continued working in this way up until the early seventies (they have always been responsible for the making of the basic salve used in our Rescue Remedy cream). When I joined Nora Weeks and Victor Bullen in 1971 (with my sister joining us from 1974 through to 1987) we were able to cope with bottling and labelling in our own right, allowing Nelsons to continue in a lesser capacity, whilst we as a team, were capable then of handling all home and overseas orders along with our other duties.

With such a long standing association with Nelsons, we decided when our new production unit was introduced, to turn to them once more to take on the full and responsible management that such a unit demanded. They were our obvious choice, in fact the only people to whom we could entrust such an important undertaking of distributing and marketing the Bach Flower Remedies. This is done under licenced agreement, under our full supervision, and Nelsons have committed themselves to upholding the standards and principles of Dr. Bach at all times.

The Mother Tinctures are of course still made by us at the Bach Centre, which means that the production unit handles only the bottling, labelling and despatch of goods – so in answer to the question, the quality of the Bach Flower Remedies continue absolutely without change in any form.

(Address of the Abingdon Unit and its function is listed on page 118)

How can 2 drops only of a Remedy do so much – surely there must be something more to it than that?

It has often been said that the simplicity of this work baffles the professionals, and people attempt to look for something that is not there. Does one question the nutritional value of a cabbage? The warming of the body from a fire when one is cold, or the refreshing coolness of the air when one is stuffy? – all such things are taken for granted and not scrutinized in any way. So, by the same token, the healing quality of a plant should be accepted, without question. Nature provides the air we breathe, the food we eat, the very essence of life itself – so who can deny that it must also provide the means to make us well! We must not forget that nearly all forms of medicine are derived originally from plant life – so there should be nothing odd or strange to behold in the healing quality of wild flowers.

Do you have failures with these Remedies, you never mention them?

As in all methods of treatment there are certain clients who fail to respond. Over a long period we have kept records of our clients and find an average of seventy-five per cent, are so much better they need no more treatment.

The failure to help the other twenty-five per cent may be attributed to the prescriber's inability to find the client's real difficulty and consequently prescribe wrongly, or it may arise from lack of perserverance on the part of the recipient, or in a few cases from a lack of real desire to get well for some private personal reason.

We have heard that there is now a Radiation Remedy – is that true?

There is a composite called 'Radiation Remedy' formulated by Dr. Aubrey Westlake – but it has to be stated quite categorically that it is not a Bach Remedy proper. Dr. Westlake clearly 'admits', when referring to the Bach Remedies in his book 'The Pattern of Health' – that in his particular view, a "... direct treatment of the physical may be needed as well", and that therefore he created the Radiation Remedy in keeping with that opinion. Dr. Westlake also fairly acknowledges that in so doing, he had 'DEPARTED FROM THE SIMPLE USE OF THE BACH REMEDIES AS TAUGHT BY DR. BACH, AND HAD INTRODUCED A MORE COMPLICATED

CONCEPT FOR USING THEM." He went further to quote from one of the Bach Centre's early News Letters, an unequivocal statement in an article by Nora Weeks and Victor Bullen, that the 38 Remedies were complete and that there was no extension to what was first conceived by Dr. Bach himself.

From the foregoing it will be gathered that Dr. Westlake was attempting a combination of Bach Remedies that he thought would generally alleviate a conditioned state created by outside forces. The Bach theory would be to consider each individual in his/her attitude to the problem of radiation fallout. One person might be full of great apprehension or terror, imagining poisons entering the system with every breath taken . . . whereas another would not feel unduly alarmed, but feel that it be sensible to take something just in case. Each of these persons would quite obviously require different remedies and it is on this basis that the Bach Remedies would be diagnosed and dispensed, with Crab Apple (the cleanser) being firmly considered for most cases.

In case anyone is interested in Dr. Westlake's preparation, it consists of a mixture of Cherry Plum, Star of Bethlehem, Rock Rose, Gentian, Vine, Walnut and Wild Oat. His recommendation is that it be prepared thus: 2 drops of each remedy to a mixture of 3.5g sea salt diluted in 100 ml of pure spring water. Dosage is exactly the same as for Rescue Remedy.

We know that Holly and Wild Oat are Dr. Bach's declared catalysts – but recently Star of Bethlehem has been added to these in some references. Can you please clear this matter up for us?

This assumption is incorrect – there are only the two (Holly and Wild Oat) as determined by Dr. Bach. It seems that the error occurs in 'The Handbook of the Bach Flower Remedies', which is a compilation of all the descriptions and case histories of each Remedy that Nora Weeks had featured systematically in her News Letters over the years. Philip Chancellor, under Nora's guidance, collated them together under the one cover, thereby producing a very worthwhille *and in depth reference* book for practitioners.

The following quotes will show that Dr. Chancellor's descriptive use of the word 'catalyst' was of his own making, as it was not included in the original News Letter wording, hence the misinterpretation and confusion.

Quote (a) – <u>News Letter Original</u>: 'In treating some cases, therefore, who do not seem to respond well, it is a good thing to keep Star of Bethlehem in mind, and to find out gently from the patient whether at any time in the recent or quite distant past he or she has suffered from some great shock or distress of mind, or disappointment.'

Quote (b) – <u>Chancellor's version of the above</u>: 'Therefore, when treating a case which does not respond to the Remedies prescribed, it is well to bear Star of Bethlehem in mind; it might be the catalyst that was lacking! Try to discover, in a most gentle manner, whether the patient has had a severe shock in his or her past life.'

For the benefit of those who need to be reminded of the

significance of the doctor's catalysts . . . they are taken whenever a case suggests that it needs many remedies or if it does not respond to treatment – the appropriate one will then help to determine the obvious correct choice of Remedies. In cases where the person is of the active, intense type, give Holly . . . and Wild Oat when the person is a weak and despondent type. (They are intended for use only as a final resort – normal prescribing should not be forsaken in the hope that the catalysts will automatically reveal in advance the remedies required).

We have often been asked to give the meaning of Dr. Bach's qualifications – they are as follows:

L.R.C.P.: Licentiate of the Royal College of Physicians.
M.R.C.S.: Member Royal College of Surgeons.
M.B.: Bachelor of Medicine.
B.S.: Bachelor of Surgery.
D.P.H.: Diploma of Public Health.

What type of man was Dr. Bach?

Many would see in Dr. Bach the epitome of a great soul in earthly guise, a person of wonderful thought, high intellect, great vision, healing qualities above the norm, profound spirtual awareness of knowledge and Truth – yet for all that, a humble man of normal habits and suffering, who accepted such adverse conditions of life as a valuable experience to the betterment of his own development.

Those of us who have experienced the wonderful gift

he bestowed upon the world through his Flower Remedies and his wise teachings will want to revere his name for all time – and so it should be. Yet – he would be the last to expect such recognition, in fact he would refuse any credit at all, for in his own eyes, he was but an instrument used by Nature and his God – he felt that he was of little consequence. Let us therefore give quiet 'thanks' for his being, but at the same time be careful that we do not over indulge his name by creating a saint-like image that would be absolutely foreign to his own wishes. Dr. Bach was as human as any other person in that he had a good sense of humour, loved to mix with the locals in the public house, for a chat, drink and sing-song. He could be irritable and sometimes difficult like any one of us, but at the same time was kind, generous (to an extreme degree, some would say) and humble. He became so intent on finalizing his work during the latter two years of his life – 'mundane' matters such as food and clothing meant very little to him. The quality of his discovery may be described as 'Divine', but in himself he was quite a character and most certainly very human.

Why did he die so young?

The question of his 'dying at such an early age' often crops up – in fact people wonder why, in being such a brilliant physician, he was not in a position to 'cure' himself. If one accepts that our real life is the soul or spirit (whichever) then 'dying' is of little consequence, no matter at what age it might take place. Death is not the end, it is only a transitional passage returning us to our natural state of being. So, as in the case of Dr. Bach, having completed his work, it was time for him to 'depart' to continue his work in other spheres.

Is it possible to make up a combination of remedies for a common condition or situation that many people suffer?

Going to the dentist; sitting examinations; auditions; speaking in public, going for an interview . . . these are but a few of the traumatic experiences we all have to suffer at different stages of our lives and how fortunate we are to have Dr. Bach's own original combination to turn to – Rescue Remedy – which had proved itself quite adequately over the years in helping people through such trying times. The question of a pre-determined combination remedy would mean trying to cater for every person's different approach to the problem, and unless one combined all 38, then it would be a very difficult task. Fear is the predominant condition – but what type of fear? Is it a great doubt in one's ability to face the situation . . . in other words a personal fear of letting oneself down . . . or perhaps the fear of how one pays the mortgage if the result of the interview or examination is not successful? Some people will be philosophical about the whole thing – 'if I fail – well . . . I'll try again', whereas another type would be in absolute dread of the outcome because of what would hinge on the result. There are those with bad memories . . . others (Scleranthus types) who would waste precious time trying to choose the right subject for an essay . . . others, normally quite capable, would find themselves being tongue-tied or their minds going blank purely through panic. Every person has to be treated uniquely – judged by *their* particular state of mind alone – one cannot generalise.

We are often asked if the Bach Remedies can be incorporated in other products, e.g. creams, herbal preparations, oils, etc.

As much as we can understand the enhancement offered, by the inclusion of the Remedies, to other preparations, regretfully we have to refuse permission for this to be done. Apart from the fact that the Remedies must remain a separate entity in their own right, the question of liability also becomes paramount. Our very heavy premiums cover the Bach product only – there is no accommodation that extends beyond that – this is one of the reasons why the Bach title (including Rescue Remedy) is protected by a trade mark, to ensure that Bach's good name is not brought into disrepute in any form through involvement with products that could be of a dubious nature. It would also be extremely unfair of us at this stage to adopt a new policy in this respect after so many refusals to genuine requests over the years . . . We feel certain that people of understanding minds will fully appreciate our position.

When choosing Remedies does one treat the positive aspect?

The positive comparisons are featured in our charts and 'Dictionary of the BFR' purely as a guide to the state one should be in *after* having dealt with the negative outlook. The answer to the question therefore is 'NO – treat only the negative'.

Practical Use of the
Remedies

A Guide to Prescribing

THERE are 38 Remedies in all, each relative to a specific state of mind. It is not unusual for a person at first, to declare the need for all 38 at the same time! This of course would not be done – not that there would be any harm in doing so, but they just don't work that way (see page 64). It is essential therefore to judge one's predominant state of mind or 'type'; determine how one reacts to certain situations or actions of other people; if there has been some emotional upset or strain, then how one becomes effected by this. Feelings of hatred, envy jealousy; or resentment leading to self pity and so on, are states of mind we all experience at times, normally being able to overcome such problems if they are only of a fleeting nature, but when such emotions begin to take root, and we become too incensed by such feelings, we do then need to adjust our thinking, otherwise we might find ourselves in a whirlpool or on a 'slope to nowhere' that can seriously effect the very pattern of our lives.

The first step is to read up on the subject (see book descriptions on pages 20–23). By making a determined study of the remedies and their related states of mind, the novice should soon be able to bring to mind automatically, the correct remedy or group of remedies that would apply when an obvious type or state of mind revealed itself (see also page 58).

Finding out why or how a particular state of mind has been created (see page 56) is of great importance – pealing the onion as we call it. If indecision is created by fear, then in treating the cause (fear) rather than the effect

45

(indecision), you are getting to the core of the problem. It might be that the indecision is deep rooted enough to warrant a remedy also, but the required basic remedy must not be omitted. Let us take the example of a gentle, generous and ever-willing lady with a widowed mother to look after. Her family had always been closely knit, the mother sacrificing a lot to ensure that she (the daughter) never went hungry or short in any way – in other words, a brave and loving person. But unfortunately, there is also a tendency of possessiveness (not recognised by the daughter because of her feeling of gratitude and love), and so the mother accepts all the daughter's kind attention, but in addition draws from her a sense of duty as her right! As time progresses, the daughter realizes that all her friends are now married and raising their own families, while she is duty-bound running up and down stairs with a tray in her hand all day. This realization brings thoughts of resentment (bordering on hatred at times) towards her mother, mental arguments galore, feelings of despondency and self detestation for thinking such thoughts which are so foreign to her basic nature. There are remedies for all these states of mind (viz. Willow, Holly, White Chestnut, Gentian, Crab Apple) – and although such remedies would lift her to a degree that she would be able to face the day that much better, the result would not be lasting because the basic 'type' remedy has not been included, and so, like the tide, all her ill feelings and doubts would return starting the cycle all over again. The 'type' to recognize here is the subservient ever willing worker, commonly known as the 'doormat', unable to say 'no' or draw the line, and the remedy for such a person is *Centaury*. With the help of this remedy, she would be able to approach her mother and say "I'm going out tonight mother" . . . the mother, acting the martyr, would look somewhat crestfallen and say (with meaning) "You go and enjoy yourself – don't worry about me, I'll be alright on my own. I don't suppose I'll be with you much longer and then I won't be a burden to you any more". Now normally this would be sufficient to make the daughter peel off her coat and remain indoors . . . but with the strength of Centaury, her individuality will have returned and she'd find herself being brave enough to give her mother a kiss, tell her that she won't be long and that Mrs. Jones downstairs will hear her if she rings her bell, and go. Now – having done it once, she can do it again – in other words she is controlling 'it' rather than 'it' controlling her, and in having revivified her status as a person in her own right, as opposed to being a slave, all the states of mind created by her past weakness would begin to dissipate – dejection, resentment and self condemnation would go (she would now begin to feel proud of herself) and so would the need for the related remedies. This is a typical case of finding the true basic essential remedy – if one or two of the other states of mind are still lingering then the additional remedy or remedies can be added – but the all important one is Centaury in this case. The mother would need Chicory!

Do you have a special way of conducting a consultation?

Our particular method is as follows. We first of all greet the client in a warm or friendly manner, invite them to

47

sit in a position that allows *you* (the interviewer) a vantage point of being within easy reach of literature, sample bottles and so on, as well as allowing yourself a 'good view' of the person's general mannerisms, expression and attitude. Depending on circumstances – a client having travelled some distance, or if we are about to have one ourselves, a cup of tea is offered – this helps to put people at their ease and feel at home. The next step, is to determine the purpose of the visit, and if it is necessary, to briefly explain the principle of this method of healing first, before proceeding further. (Many people are quite knowledgeable, whereas others know very little concerning Dr. Bach and his work, and do welcome some enlightenment on the subject).

Once we get down to the matter of helping the client – we then allow he or she to tell us in their own words the purpose of their visit – if it flows in keeping with what we would require to know, we would then only interject when necessary to determine or enlarge on an important fact mentioned. Whilst this is going on we would be ticking up particular remedies on our consultation pad, in keeping with what we were learning from the discourse. Eventually, we would have the basis of the person's remedy requirement and by the process of elimination, again through pertinent questions, would narrow the choice down to a reasonable number of approximately six remedies, or less. Some people are extremely easy to determine and an interview can be over within 15 minutes or so, whereas others can be more 'difficult', and it is then up to us to delve more deeply, not only by questioning, but perhaps by open discussion concerning the person's home life, hobbies, work. If there is a certain reticence or inability to communicate with the standard suggestions put forward, the less formal discussion about home life and work will often dislodge the basic hidden problem behind the person's stress or worry. Without realising its significance, he (the client) might disclose the fact that life at work could be very good indeed, but it was becoming intolerable because of *'that stupid idiot of a boss who just cannot appreciate anything worthwhile ... still it doesn't worry me'*. brave words maybe – but here is what we needed to know – this is the heart of the matter. Treatment is then based on how he faces up to this frustration or annoyance ... if he hides it and pretends it doesn't exist, not wanting others to see him 'bothered' with such problems, and brushes it off with a grin – then he basically needs Agrimony. Obviously if his thoughts haunted him and hatred towards his boss was welling up inside him, then White Chestnut and Holly respectively would suggest themselves (along with others perhaps). If on the other hand he was very subservient and ran around in circles to try and please and appease his manager then Centaury would be called for ... and so it could go on.

It must be said of course, that our knowledge over the years has been gained through our association with Nora Weeks who taught us all that we needed to know. Getting to thoroughly *know* the remedies is of prime importance ... Dr. Bach's description of each is so specific, and easy to understand, yet the profundity of his findings put together in a simple nutshell is a feat of engineering in itself, for it offers a knowledge of human nature to a degree of such proportions, that Psychiatrists have scratched their heads in absolute astonishment, because it presents a level of expertise equal to that which they have only attained after years and years of study.

Dr. Bach listed two essentials that a healer must bear in mind – first to encourage the person's individuality, and the second to teach him to look ahead – in other words raise their confidence and hope.

One thing we learn for certain, and that is the wonderful rapport that builds up between our clients and ourselves – this proves the importance of allowing a worried man, a frantic or frightened lady to open up and shed their problems in absolute confidence and trust. This is a therapy in itself, in their having an understanding ear and compassionate adviser to turn to. It astounds them to think that we 'know them' better than they perhaps know themselves – this engenders a beautiful trust, not only in what they hope we can do for them, but in the actual remedies themselves. To see people depart in a happy frame of mind with faith in their ability to change for the better irrespective of their problem is wonderful to behold.

Every case is separate, and must be treated as such. Some are fairly easy, others more complex, but nevertheless the challenge is a very enjoyable one, which can only be experienced fully by prescribing the remedies in the intended manner – through Dr. Bach's basic method.

How long does one have to take the Remedies before obtaining some result?

There are many ways to answer this – a great deal depends on how deep rooted is the actual problem itself. If one wakes up one day with a typical 'Monday morning' feeling, then a couple of drops of Hornbeam in a small glass of water, sipped whilst getting oneself ready for work should then do the trick. A feeling of apprehension or foreboding would be helped in the same way with Aspen. This form of treatment deals with the ups and downs of every-day living, changing moods, etc., but when it comes to a much more long-standing problem, then further details are necessary before determining the basic or type remedy.

Let us take the common see-saw as a sample image to illustrate what we mean:–

Fig. 1.

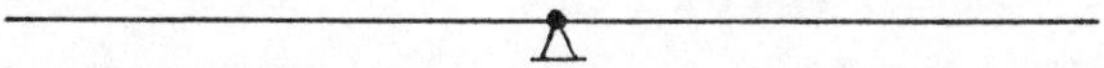

Fig. 1 shows the see-saw levelled at an even keel. This is the equilibrium that represents us in our natural state, allowing us to progress through life, tackling all the lessons and experiences laid out in our paths before us – it is coming through these conditions successfully that enable us to climb our ladder of evolution . . . but few of us manage to complete all our tasks without some struggle or deviation to slow us down, or send us off on a tangent . . . and that is where the Remedies come into their own, to help us re-adjust.

Let us take as an example, a man who is quite capable and enjoys his work thoroughly – he is continuing along, at this stage, at an even keel. One day he finds that the success of his business brings with it a lot more responsibility, and this he feels is beginning to weigh rather heavily on his mind . . . FIG. 2 REPRESENTS THE TILT TO HIS EQUILIBRIUM thus slowing down his progress (position A).

Fig. 2.   A

. . . at this early stage, the roots have not taken hold, and so the adjustment at the central point of balance is very slight – in other words, the appropriate Remedy Elm, if taken at this moment would act as a preventative/prophylactic, and the balance would very soon return to the normal level, and so progress would continue again as before.

BUT, if he were to allow the tilt to remain, by doing nothing to prevent the sense of inadequacy taking hold, the sequence would then produce a snowballing effect, causing him to doubt his own ability (whereas previously he was full of confidence), – this in turn could lead to fears concerning the future, his home, and his family. (Positions A & C respectively – Fig 3).

Fig. 3.

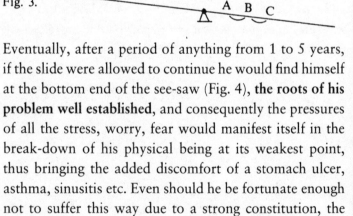

Eventually, after a period of anything from 1 to 5 years, if the slide were allowed to continue he would find himself at the bottom end of the see-saw (Fig. 4), **the roots of his problem well established**, and consequently the pressures of all the stress, worry, fear would manifest itself in the break-down of his physical being at its weakest point, thus bringing the added discomfort of a stomach ulcer, asthma, sinusitis etc. Even should he be fortunate enough not to suffer this way due to a strong constitution, the break-down would then probably be mental (position D).

Fig. 4.

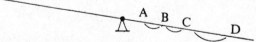

CONCLUSION: The time therefore it takes for the Remedies to have a positive effect can be judged by the position one might be at, on the slide – the deeper you are, the greater the angle of correction. It is important to realise that treatment for a person at the bottom of the see-saw would still be the same as at stage A, because that was the basic reason for the initial breakdown. Other predominant conditions that have built up would also be considered, along with the 'type' remedy if significant. Another point to remember – when looking at the tilted see-saw don't mistakenly think that because the lower side is the negative, that the highest point automatically represents the positive – that would be wrong. When one adjusts the negative, the opposite end returns downwards from the apex to the same even keel forming the HAPPY MEDIUM – *that* is the true positive state.

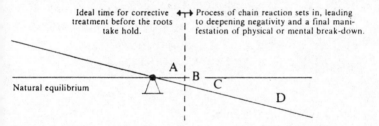

Ideal time for corrective treatment before the roots take hold.

Process of chain reaction sets in, leading to deepening negativity and a final manifestation of physical or mental break-down.

Natural equilibrium

A B C D

One of your earlier New Letters suggested certain Remedies for particular groups of recognisable people – one such group were those subjected to tyrranical control, with no hope of escape – namely 'Galley Slaves'. My question is would your suggested remedies help such souls to accept the situation meakly, or in fact invoke them to rise up and smash the chains that bind them? (Hypothetical maybe – but interesting)

This question offers us the chance perhaps to explain how the Remedies bring the sufferer to a state of happy medium (an even keel) by actually finding the course between the two extremes.

People subjected to tyranny, if they are of hope and courage will show measured restraint and break the chains **when the time is right for them to do so.** But probably the majority would be completely subjugated to the point of acceptance of their lot, without even a flicker of hope, their 'strength' shut off under the blanket effect of total rule. Such attributes as individuality, ego, thought, decision, can, with the help of the Remedies, be rekindled, not necessarily to bring about an uprising, but to return self esteem and awareness and strength to their inner selves, so that progression will start to take place once more, and the experience and subjection can then be 'accepted' in a positive sense. 'Acceptance' in this light is an essential part of learning showing the true purpose of the restriction and fortifying the faith that carries one through to eventual and 'inevitable' release.

What is a 'Type' Remedy?

The 'type' is determined by the basic fundamental nature of a person – the personality trait or temperament that is 'natural' or innate. Some Remedies are complementary or helpers and often need to be given to back-up a basic type remedy. It must be remembered though that type remedies do have a wider connotation and can be used at times as a helper. For example – Scleranthus deals with the types who can never make up their minds one way or the other – yet it also helps those who suffer fluctuating moods or some form of imbalance, irrespective of type.

It is equally important to analyse one's initial choice of

remedies – especially if they total something like 10 or 12 in number. By a process of elimination, working backwards, one will find a common denominator that represents the truly required 'type', or, basic remedy or group of remedies that present the probables from your original list of possibles. There is a state of cause and effect in the mind as well as between mind and body – so if you melt down the emotional snow-ball that has developed – then the real choice of remedies will become much clearer. (see also page 64)

(P.S. Examples of basic 'types' are: Agrimony, Centaury, Cerato, Chicory, Clematis, Heather, Impatiens, Larch, Mustard, Oak, Pine, Rock Water, Scleranthus, Vervain, Vine, Water Violet. Some of the remaining Remedies are 'grey area', with others being created by circumstances and conditions or simply acting as helper remedies, e.g. Olive, White Chestnut, Hornbeam).

Can a remedy be given without the recipient knowing, and if so is it morally right?

People can be treated this way – and very successfully. The remedies can be detected in water and any beverage containing milk . . . so the best means of administering is in fruit juice or liquor. If the Bach Remedies were harmful, we would certainly not consider it ethical to treat anyone without permission, but the wonderful help a person can receive by this natural and benign treatment is akin to offering them your love, which most of us would still continue to give even if it were shunned or ridiculed. The same criterion is used in giving the remedies without consent. A person no doubt would be pleased to learn afterwards how they had been helped.

Dr. Bach said that each of the 38 remedies cover every state of mind known to man . . . but surely there must be more than 38 states of mind . . . e.g. you don't relate to anger, boredom, or anxiety specifically?

Such conditions as stated above represent sub-headings – they are states of mind that can be caused or created by any manner of related problems. So it is all important to begin by determing 'How?' or 'Why?' any predominant condition of mind manifests itself. Anger is often associated with hatred and envy, which would immediately suggest Holly – but – that is by no means a final prognosis, because anger can be equally caused by frustration, worry, resentment or any other conditioned state of mind – so the final choice has to be determined by finding out the basic cause behind the anger. Similarly, worry, fear, anxiety, depression would need further 'investigation' before determining the correct Remedy. Lack of concentration can be due to many different states – boredom, tiredness, pre-occupied mind, lethargy, lack of confidence, escapism, laziness, fear, etc., each with their own related remedy or composition of remedies. So, in coming down to basics, there *are* only 38 states to consider. Working in composites (many people require more than the one remedy in the one preparation) will extend the possible permutation of required remedies into a much wider spectrum of choice.

Take another example – a man and wife might both complain of being anxious – yet on investigation it would be found that he, although normally a capable man, was beginning to feel inadequate due to the pressure of responsibility at work, whereas his wife was over concerned about the welfare of their son. Their respective treatments would be entirely different – he would need Elm, whereas she Red Chestnut, yet both suffered the same state of mind!

I notice that Dr. Bach lists 3 particular remedies under the heading 'Loneliness' in his 'Twelve Healers' . . . does a lonely person therefore take these 3 remedies?

No . . . Dr. Bach's seven headings represent a classification of certain types that correlate generally under his respective headings. In the case of 'Loneliness' he lists Water Violet, Impatiens and Heather – the first two represent types who *prefer* to be alone of their own choosing. The third remedy is for the person who seeks out company for the sole (and rather selfish) purpose of talking for the sake of talking (mostly about their own ailments and problems!). It will be gathered therefore, that when those who are thrust into loneliness, by events of circumstances, then one seeks out the appropriate remedy. For example – a shy timid, fearful person is often very lonely, and it would be basically Mimulus that this person would require.

Can treatment bottles be used more than once?

Yes indeed – boil the bottle, black screw cap and glass pipette for 10 to 20 minutes – then dry in a heated oven (this prevents the formation of white residue on the glass).

The rubber teat can be dipped in boiling water and squeezed out to clean the inner part . . . but this part does not actually come in contact with any remedy normally, so the quick dip should suffice.

Would the Centre appreciate having empty bottles returned to them?

At one time when there was a glass shortage we would certainly have welcomed them, but with that particular problem no longer causing us concern, we prefer now to use fresh bottles for our new orders and treatments. The volume of work has reached such a pitch nowadays that returned bottles would slow us down considerably due to the huge sterilisation programme we would have to adopt. Thank you for the thought nevertheless.

How can I get to know the Remedies better other than by reading the books?

First of all, it is quite obvious that the Remedies and their respective states of mind must be thoroughly learned, so that any suitable Remedy will automatically spring to mind when the appropriate condition becomes known. Learn them as you would the Morse Code so that you get an immediate reaction in your mind. Having mastered this you will then find many opportunities to put not only your memory, but your intuitive powers to the test. The quiet study of people around you at work and at parties, will offer an advanced degree of perception. But, for beginners, the theatre and television present an untapped source of characterisations – all over-emphasized, because in play acting the character portrayals need to be pronounced to satisfy the dimentional requirement of entertainment. So you see, you can turn your TV viewing time into a worthwhile occupation for a change. You'll be surprised how often you will begin to associate the Remedies with various personalities, characters, and types portrayed. Practise on willing friends and members of the family – it can be quite fun.

I have heard of people suffering reactions after taking the remedies – can you explain this please?

First of all it is important to know that the Remedies do not create any adverse condition. If a person develops a rash for example, this, as far as the Bach Remedies are concerned would be a positive step, representing the cleansing of toxins from the system. The same would apply to states of mind that might appear to the sufferer, to be 'quite foreign to one's normal pattern of thought'. Some people bury certain emotional feelings in their sub-conscious – they don't like the particular thought they are experiencing and mentally swallow it – thus the lesson of such an emotion has not been fully gained. Therefore it stands to reason, that before any cure can be effected, the cleansing has to take place and so the toxins or deep rooted emotions have to pass through and out of one's system, an 'effect' that should not be of long duration. This is a release to be welcomed. It is often said that 'one cannot get out what is not already there' or 'you cannot stir a muddy pool without bringing the silt to the surface'. One point to appreciate is that any such reaction is not a side effect – it is your own mind or body correcting itself aided and abetted by the Remedies.

Can the stock concentrate remedies be taken undiluted?

If liquid is totally unavailable, then the drops can be taken direct from the stock bottle, but it must be remembered that the preservative is undiluted brandy and therefore abstainers must be warned of this fact – it would be very irresponsible of us not to consider alcoholics or people who, on religious grounds would not wish alcohol to pass their lips. It is always better that the remedies be diluted if only in a spoonful of water, which is then held in the mouth for a few moments, and as one swallows, try to imagine it as a cleansing light invading the whole system, driving out the 'darkness' of the condition from which one might be suffering. We do state that if a person is in a comatose state, then the application of Rescue Remedy (undiluted if necessary) can be applied to the temples, wrists, behind the ears, or to the lips – this is purely an emergency method of applying the remedy when it is impracticable to administer in drink form. Taking remedies direct from a concentrate bottle does not enhance the strength of the dosage – 2 drops in water are equally effective, of any individual remedy, or 4 drops of Rescue Remedy.

How can the remedies help people who are considered to be 'incurable' and thus condemned to a life time of suffering?

We have always upheld the belief that suffering, of any kind, be it physical or mental, will not be 'cured' if a person is *intended* (through suffering) to gain a lesson or experience essential to their own higher development. This does not mean that a person has to be condemned to the shocking finality of 'There is nothing more I can do for you – you will have to live with this' . . . no, indeed not, the Remedies can be used to raise the person's hope and revivify their faith that there *is a definite purpose to*, and chance to overcome their suffering. This new found positive outlook allows progression to take place once more (for the experience might only be short, who can tell) and in the right frame of mind a balance between mind and body takes place, thus allowing the body to heal itself naturally as it is intended. Referring to people who took the remedies prior to passing-on – Nora Weeks would remark "Well they at least died happy!" (Humerous in its way, but nevertheless very true.)

If during the course of taking a treatment mixture, another emotional characteristic becomes apparent is it alright to mix another lot separately and take them as well, but at different times?

No, it is not necessary to make up another bottle, simply add the particular remedy required to the existing one – then, when you are ready to make up a fresh bottle, you can discard those that have done their work, and stick to the fresh prescription.

Is it necessary to make up a treatment bottle even for only one state of mind that might appear one morning?

If someone wakes up with a feeling of apprehension/foreboding, or perhaps impatience, or even the common 'Monday morning' feeling, then an appropriate remedy (2 drops in a glass of water and sipped at intervals whilst preparing oneself before leaving) can be taken accordingly. It is not necessary to prepare a dosage bottle that would last normally about 3 weeks, for such everyday mood flucuations.

When would I stop taking the remedies . . . and what would result if I continued beyond the need?

When one feels a definite betterment, it is then that one can stop taking the remedies . . . but don't be afraid to continue with the appropriate remedies should a mood or state of mind develop at any time. As they are harmless, the time factor is not important, especially as they are not employed as a 'course' of treatment. It is a very individual approach, one suits oneself and oneself only. An indication of improvement is when one forgets to take them (!), the interest and attention having been diverted from the self flowing outward instead of inward.

Another example – an intolerant person treated with Beech, would soon begin to see good qualities in other people – this would be the positive outlook, and by natural choice one would wish to remain in this more pleasant state. This is when the remedies have completed their work, because the person has become his 'real self' again.

If one did continue with the remedies when they were no longer needed, they would simply have no effect . . . so there would be no cause for worry on this score at all – this would apply even should the wrong remedy be taken.

For how long should one continue with the same remedy if no improvement is felt, before changing it for another?

Continue with the remedy for at least a fortnight, and then if no improvement is felt in any way, represcribe. If some slight progress has been made, however small, continue with that remedy and add another or others, that might be applicable.

Can one become immune or 'used to' the remedies in that they can no longer offer their wonderful healing qualities.

The simple answer – NO. With the taking of drugs the body creates a tolerance level by natural adjustment which increases when the threshold is reached . . . antibodies are similarly built up to counteract foreign organisms (viz. germs). There is absolutely no need for the body to react or create any antidotal system when taking the Bach Remedies. Also, they are not habit-forming, in fact the very reverse, because, in spite of oneself, greater strength and self reliance develops and the need for the Remedies diminishes – they are constructive, not destructive, and most certainly are not palliatives.

If the remedies are harmless and one does not negate the other – why then can I not take all 38 remedies at once to ensure that I take the right ones? Your literature suggests no more than 6 at the one time, can you explain the contradiction?

We can fully understand the confusion due to what might appear to be conflicting statements. In answer to the question proper, Dr. Bach made a point of testing out a composite of all 38 Remedies and was not satisfied with the result. The suggestion of up to 6 remedies is meant only as a guide line – it is not a stipulation. It should not be difficult to limit one's choice to within this number – but if by chance your prescribed list extends to 7 or 8, and to reduce this number might bring about the omission of one of the essential remedies – then it is better to include them all . . . but in time, experience will help you to develop a means of being more selective. The less clouded the choice, the fairer one is, in allowing the essential remedies to do their work that much better. If an individual is typical of a particular type then the one obvious Remedy would restore the balance, whereas another (and this is the general trend) would be more complex and require a mixture of remedies to deal with the various negative aspects that are predominant – and although at first glance quite a lot of remedies might appear to be necessary, with a little study one would reduce the number to a sensible proportion. It is important to ask the question 'Why?' . . . why am I tense, depressed, afraid, unhappy, confused, weak etc? – the resulting answers if honestly assessed would produce a basic reason. Remember 'cause and effect' – if for instance a person suffers uncertainty because of fear – then treat the fear and the uncertainty would go too! (see general instructions at end of chapter).

If two Remedies diametrically opposed are put in the same treatment bottle, do they cancel each other out?

The answer is no – they do not negate each other. If a person was a 'Vine type' (of determined views who would rule rather than serve), then giving him the remedy for the subservient character (Centaury) would have no effect whatsoever other than to cloud the issue a little – *unless of course* there was a peripheral need at the time, e.g. if some habit enslaved him or perhaps he became 'putty' in the hands of a person of the opposite sex!

Is it possible to take homoeopathic remedies at the same time as the Bach Remedies?

Despite the sensitivity of certain Homoeopathic medicines – many homoeopathic doctors do prescribe the Bach Remedies. The Bach Remedies will neither interfere with, nor be affected by, any other form of medicinal treatment.

If I were a person not prone to lose my temper, be angry or intolerant – would it be sensible for me to take the appropriate remedies to protect myself from ever becoming intolerant etc?

One does not take remedies in advance of states of mind *that might be created* . . . obviously you can take those that will cater for the mental worry, apprehension or fear that might be building up towards the event, but you would not take a remedy as a precautionary measure as suggested in the question – you would only take the remedy should such a state of mind manifest itself, to make the adjustment before it begins to take root. There would be no point whatsoever in a determined person, who knows his own mind, taking SCLERANTHUS as a safeguard against indecision. If doubt began to creep in, making him lose the ability to make up his mind, *then* he would turn to that particular remedy.

We understand that some people are suggesting that the opposite remedy be taken to strengthen the positive aspect of a person. For example – if the person were the weak subservient gentle type (CENTAURY) – the taking of Vine would enhance the strength that that person needed – *this is absolutely wrong* – it is the *Centaury Remedy* that brings about the positive aspect in such people, because it helps them to say 'No' when necessary, to prevent advantage being taken of their kind natures, by the more forceful and demanding personalities. The positive state of a Centaury type does not mean a changed personality – they remain the same generous and willing people as they were always intended to be, but capable of controlling the situation properly, when it affects them, with a gentle strength of will.

Can the description of one person given by another be sufficient and satisfactory when prescribing?

A lot depends on how well they know each other. Usually a man or wife can describe the state and outlook of the spouse quite well ... but one must be wary of for instance, the 'ruler' of the family trying to describe the sensitivity of his or her partner. Usually such a powerful nature would condemn the other as a weak and easily led person not realising the real fault for this lay in their own aggressive and ruling manner (in which case they too should be treated to help bring about a deeper understanding of the true value of gentle sincerity and generosity of spirit embodied in his or her partner). Nevertheless, the prescriber would, for the weaker person, still recognize basically the need for Centaury.

Often there is little choice in the matter – lethargy, shyness, doubt, illness or some other difficult circumstance might prevent direct contact – so it is up to the practitioner to be very discerning, and to ask the right questions to find out just what is required to be known about the other person. Usually close friends and parents can give quite a valuable assessment of those for whom they seek help. One consolation is that if we are wrongly advised then the incorrect choice of remedies would do no harm, and it would then be a pointer to our need for a more accurate description.

You suggest pure spring water in your dosage instructions – can you clarify this please?

Spring water can be purchased in health food stores or supermarkets – it needs to be the non-gas type to prevent a gassy overflow when filling the treatment bottle. Distilled water is not recommended because it is a 'dead' liquid, it is devoid of natural properties.

COMPARISONS

There is a very thin dividing line sometimes separating the choice between certain remedies of similar ilk – this brings doubt and concern to the less experienced prescriber.

The following comparisons might elucidate further:–

What is the difference between Larch, Scleranthus and Cerato? They all seem to indicate lack of confidence.

LARCH people lack confidence in their ability to do things – they expect to fail and so make no attempt. They have the ability but due to fear of failure (and success for that matter) they would prefer to stand back in the shadow and allow others, even of lesser talent, to take their place. Self consciousiness enters into it – and the support of a 'fear remedy' is often needed.

SCLERANTHUS folk are torn btween the choice of two things – find it difficult to say 'yes' or 'no' – always caught in two minds. Vacillation, indecision are the key words. They struggle to find the answer themselves – they do not seek help from others.

CERATO is indicated for people who know their own minds, can make decisions, but when made, do not trust them, so seek the advice (seeking confirmation) of others. They are inclined to be persistent in their demand for others' opinions. The problem really is that they do not have confidence in their own judgement.

What is the difference between the tiredness of Hornbeam and Olive?

HORNBEAM people are those who suffer the perpetual 'Monday morning feeling' – they are uncertain whether they have the strength to face the day, yet once started they find that they are quite able to carry on. The tiredness is more in the mind than the body – it is just a matter of getting started.

OLIVE is the remedy for those who have gone through long periods of mental difficulties or responsibilities or worries, or are perhaps recovering from a painful or wearing illness of long duration. Mind and body are utterly weary, exhausted – there is no vitality left to make any effort, life has lost its zeal. Olive can help after an exhausting day that leaves you absolutely drained.

. . . Wild Rose and Clematis?

WILD ROSE is for those who accept their lot in life – they become apathetic with no set ambition – they don't worry very much about what might happen to them – 'if it's going to happen it will happen'!

CLEMATIS is for the day-dreamer, the person who lives in a different world either by reflecting constantly on fantasies or for escaping reality (find it hard to come down to earth).

Crab Apple, apart from being a 'cleanser' also relates to self condemnation – how does this compare with the guilt complex of Pine?

CRAB APPLE is taken when people feel self disgust for any reason – they look in the mirror and call themselves names, they just don't like themselves due to obesity, foolishness, bad habits, general appearance and so on.

PINE covers the people who feel guilty not only for their own mistakes, but are even prepared to blame themselves for the short-comings of others. Very apologetic – feels unworthy.

Envy and jealousy (Holly) is very close to resentment (Willow) – how does one make the choice?

HOLLY: Envy and jealousy are usually quite discernable in a person – one's verbal attitude is very indicative of feelings in this respect.

WILLOW on the other hand helps people who feel that life has been very unfair, they have a very big chip on their shoulders and become embittered about fate serving them so badly. 'Poor me' attitude is very predominant.

. . . Walnut and Honeysuckle?

WALNUT relates to those people who need to break from past influences and who are unable to adjust themselves to new surroundings or conditions of life. Any change whether physical (puberty, menopause) or through marriage, divorce, new employment, moving house etc. will be helped if the transition is not easy.

HONEYSUCKLE is for those who mentally *want to live* in the past. Nostalgia – homesickness. People can be enslaved by the past, through unpleasant happenings or regret, equally as much as by pleasurable thoughts of happy days gone by.

Can you describe the difference between the 'hopeless' Remedies – viz. Gentian, Gorse, Sweet Chestnut?

There are three stages of hopelessness:

GENTIAN is the first where despondency sets in . . . 2 steps forward and 1 back which causes doubt and discouragement.

GORSE comes next when one feels that nothing is going to help them – 'I'll try it if you say so, but I don't suppose it will do any good' or 'Oh! What's the use' are typical feeling under this category.

SWEET CHESTNUT is the final state when there is nothing but oblivion ahead – utter despair, anguish and feeling utterly alone.

What is the subtle difference between Mimulus and Aspen – both 'fear Remedies'?

MIMULUS is for fear of *known* things – fear of all the hazards of every-day living. It is also for those who are afraid or nervous of demanding situations like speaking in public, having to face crowds (this creates timidity/ shyness). Fear of any definite thing.

ASPEN is for the *unknown* fears – that bring about apprehension, foreboding. Usually people cannot speak of such fears because they cannot explain them.

What is the difference in the domineering aspect of the Vervain and Vine characters?

VERVAIN people are full of enthusiasm for the ideas and principles which they hold at the moment. They hold on to these ideas with all their might and are so sure that they would benefit others that they try hard to convert them. The idea may become too fixed and possess them, becoming 'bees in their bonnet', and, as they have strong wills, will result in tension and strain affecting bodily health. They will not give in but struggle on, forcing themselves beyond their physical strength. They would die for a cause, be burnt at the stake or suffer much for they have great courage when they are confident they are doing right. They 'live on their nerves', as it were, and are highly strung (in this they differ from the more solid Vine). Everything they do is to excess – they tend to talk a great deal, are over-tense, over-active, over-enthusiastic. They are the reformers and the converts.

VINE types are of strong character who consider they know best what is good for others. They do not try to convert others to their way of thinking, but will 'lay down the law', force others to do their will, and expect obedience. They have great capabilities, are sure of themselves, keep their head in emergencies and have determination – all excellent qualities if they do not use them to interfere with others. But their strong, forceful nature, tends to sap the confidence of others, and prevents their using their own initiative, for they insist that things should be done their way. When ill they will still direct even those caring for them and instruct them how things should be done.

Once they can overcome the desire to dominate and be

the slave-driver, they become fine characters indeed. They have great wisdom and knowledge, understanding and certainty, and are able to advise and help others by strengthening their own confidence and ability. They become wise rulers, and wise leaders.

Being critical of others seems to apply to Beech and Impatiens – can you explain how they differ in this respect?

BEECH people lack understanding, judge others by their own standards forgetting that each one of us has a different path to tread, a different way of thinking, of acting. Instead of looking for the good in those around him, he will make no allowances, will find nothing to praise, will only see the worst. The positive aspect is one of the finest qualities of all – tolerance and understanding of the difficulties of others, and the ability to see the good in everyone and everything.

The IMPATIENS character is so quick in thought and action that he becomes impatient and irritable with those who are slow. He does not like to be hindered in his work by others who cannot keep up with his own speed and for that reason he prefers to work alone. He is impatient but not intolerant, his irritability and temper may flare up quickly, but as quickly subside.

PREPARATION AND DIRECTIONS

The efficacy of the remedies will remain constant indefinitely but we cannot vouch for the life of the brandy preservative therein. They can be taken by people of all ages – there is no danger of an over-dose or side effects, and should the wrong choice be made no harm will ensue. They will not be influenced by, nor will they effect any form of medicine prescribed to a person.

First determine the personality and temperament; fears, worries, anguish and the subsequent effect in outlook and attitude. More than one remedy can be taken at the one time, but it should not be difficult to limit your choice to within six.

For travelling, long established, deep rooted problems, and treating others:

DIRECTIONS: Put 2 drops from each chosen remedy into a bottle aprox. 30ml (1 fl.oz.) capacity and fill up with Natural Spring Water* (non-gas) and take 4 drops in a tea-spoonful of water, as often as needed, but *at least* 4 times a day, especially first and last thing daily. If preferred, one can take the drops on the tongue directly from the bottle, but try to avoid contact with the glass pipette for hygienic reasons. Such a prepared dosage bottle will remain fresh for about 3 weeks if stored in a cool place, ('fridge in very warm climates). If only tap water is available, this can be boiled before use, otherwise include a spoonful of brandy or cider vinegar to the preparation to preserve the water content. Dosage drops can be added to a baby's bottle or taken in fruit juice. (Note: If during the course of taking a treatment bottle a new condition arises, the appropriate remedy can be added and when it is time to make up a fresh bottle, discard those that have done their work and continue with the fresh prescription.)

For fluctuating moods and 'ups and downs' of everyday living:

Take the required drops in a cup of water, fruit juice, or any beverage, and sip fairly frequently – replenish cup to continue treatment if need be. (Examples Hornbeam for 'Monday morning' feeling. Impatiens if irritable or impatient; Olive after a hard fatiguing day, etc.)

Taking drops in a glass of water which will last perhaps 1 day does not differ, from a point of efficacy, to having 2 drops in a treatment bottle that will last approx. 3 weeks – as long as dosage is taken at least 4 x day, that is the essential factor.

Literature and issued instructions are self-explanatory, making it quite simple for sufferers to help themselves and others. If further advice is then required a brief word picture is needed of a person's personality, temperament, general outlook, worries, etc., and reasons for same if any. Any great disappointment or upset which might have left its mark, and what effect it has had on your thoughts, actions, outlook and so on.

Please remember – consider the person's attitude of mind, feelings, worries, indecision, timidity, vexations, resentment, possessiveness, hopelessness, lethargy, hatred, overpowering or demanding nature, intolerance, tenseness, etc., and most essentially the reason 'why' there is apprehension, worry and fear, for only then will the correct remedy(s) be determined – physical conditions are only considered as a guide to the person's state of suffering and its subsequent effect on the sufferer's outlook.

It is up to the person to take medical advice if necessary.

Can you describe the uses of the Rescue Remedy Cream?

It is essentially of course an external application. The base cream itself is made by Nelsons the Homoeopathic Company – we supply them with the Rescue Remedy tincture plus Crab Apple (the cleanser) and they make up and tube the RR Cream for us (an operation that is somewhat beyond our capabilities at this time). It will interest people to learn that the cream does not contain animal fats and that in fact, honey is part of the make-up of the basic cream, which is of course, recognized as a great healer in itself.

The RR cream has a wide range of uses – it has proved so helpful for sprains, stings, bumps, bruises, sores, burns . etc ... Often in massage the cream is applied not as a lubricant, but to act as a healing agent before manipulation. It is also used very widely in the field of sport – even those who decide to take some physical exercise not normally performed e.g. running or playing tennis – application of the cream before the event to the areas that will suffer, should help to reduce the friction that usually causes so much subsequent discomfort as a consequence of 'over-doing it'. Rescue Remedy liquid can also be applied externally, sometimes perhaps before applying the RR cream (see directions sheet).

It has often been said of the **RR Cream** – 'If in doubt – use it!'

For Those Adversely
Affected By Alcohol

———————————————

Can ALCOHOLICS be helped by the Remedies?

Because the Remedies are preserved in brandy, this naturally brings forth the questions of doubt in relation to administering them to alcoholics. First of all, as will be appreciated, the minimal drops of remedy taken in a glass of water makes the actual alcohol consumption virtually non existent, but nevertheless, that does not remove the psychological aspect even though there is no discernible taste (especially in fruit juice). Bearing this in mind, it then falls on the person concerned to weigh up the balance between the value of the treatment and our use of brandy perservative. As far as *active* alcoholics are concerned, then the Remedies can be taken in their actual drink! **Agrimony** should be considered as a probable first choice for drug addicts and alcoholics because their original facade of pretending all is well, began at some point to wear thin, and only some stimulant would offer the means of keeping up such a 'pretence'. *This diagnosis does not generally apply of course,* as for example people in a hopeless state, or those who try to escape their responsibilities would also, when the pressure is too great, seek some form of crutch or solace by the means of some false buoyancy – so different remedies would need to be considered in such cases.

The following is an excerpt from a letter written by an alcoholic that reflects very much what has just been stated and we thank him very much for his contribution:

". . . The 'type' remedy for most alcoholics will be **Agrimony**, although each person needs to be carefully tested to check this. Alcoholics are basically 'cheerful and care-free' even though by the time chronic alcoholism has set in, they are usually very depressed and morose. Someone once described my face as a picture of pain contorted into a grin, and this sums up many alcoholics, striving to keep a brave face while at the same time being tortured by life's problems . . . rather like the mask of a clown with a smile painted on his face forever keeping those jokes flowing, with no one knowing what lay behind the mask. **Agrimony** will help you to work out your problems in a joyful way – in my experience there will be a lot of laughs too, which is really what we alcoholics are after!"

Drug Addicts: As with alcoholics (diagnosis is very similar), the need for some form of crutch, escapism or stimulation is sought by the user. To treat them with the Bach Remedies, one has to determine if possible certain facts:–

(a) What was the reason for taking the drugs in the first place? . . . (e.g. boredom, inability to face reality or responsibility, fear, conforming to outside influences, being at the end of one's tether/rope, lack of control, worry, hopelessness etc. etc.)

(b) What was the person's type, personality, temperament *before* the need for drugs arose – and in what way did the person react to the stress, worry, fear, frustration or whatever, that created the habit?

Obtain the answers to these questions and a good start will have been made in finding appropriate Remedies to help return the person to the path of final recovery

(In some ways, smoking, over-eating/indulgence, and

other such habitual pursuits can be considered in a similar way to the above method of diagnosing).

If one has an allergy to alcohol, or is an abstainer, when even the minute dose is not acceptable, is there any way to overcome such a dilemma?

It is exceedingly difficult to find an answer to this problem – it is not unlike a person in need of fish oil who cannot for certain reasons eat fish. Our remedies originate with the Mother Tinctures that need to be stored for a long period, and for this reason are preserved in an equal amount of brandy. A precise number of drops of Mother Tincture is then added to pure brandy to form the Stock Remedy from which a person can prepare a composite treatment bottle. This composite bottle would consist of but 2 drops in water – which to some would *still* represent an intake of alcohol, albeit an infinitesimal amount.

The only 'solution' therefore was to grant A. Nelson & Co., the right to produce Rescue Remedy in tablet form, but it must be pointed out that this method of preparation does involve the use of the Bach Remedies (as prepared by us) initially.

When a treatment bottle is prepared, there is no need to add alcohol to preserve the water content if one uses natural spring water (available in supermarkets). This extra additive was needed before bottled water was available because tap water has no lasting quality. Should a preservative be needed, then cider vinegar can help to this end.

If a solution is found at some future date (we are conscious of the need to find an answer) then it will be announced in our News Letter.

Those who for some reason cannot swallow liquids have found that Rescue Remedy applied externally to the wrists, temples and behind the ears has proved to be helpful – perhaps this method might act as a helpful alternative method of taking the remedies.

Pregnancy, Babies and Children

MOTHERS-TO-BE

PREGNANCY as a condition, is common to most women, but the experience itself can be entirely personal. Whether the delivery be a joyous or fearful experience, or as in the case of some women, an oft repeated 'routine', the mother-to-be is subjected, in varying degrees to shock and change, physiologically and mentally

We are often asked if the Remedies can be of help to pregnant women in overcoming their emotional suffering and apprehensions (where it applies), and the answer is a resounding 'yes' – for both pre and post natal periods.

The two factors common to most i.e. reaction and change, can be treated by the taking of Rescue Remedy and Walnut as a basic composite. In addition, each person will differ to some degree in their general attitude and so appropriate Remedies can be added accordingly where necessary, basing the choice on the predominant fear, apprehension, brave front, resignation, etc. that is apparent.

The treatment can be continued during delivery, and most essentially afterwards for some period. The mother will appreciate that in neutralising her own negative thoughts and feelings, she will prevent any such influence reaching her child, thus allowing the baby's natural equilibrium to be maintained.

External application of the Rescue Remedy might prove beneficial generally to mother and child. Under urgent or extreme circumstances the RR liquid (slightly diluted in case the child's skin might be sensitive to the brandy preservative therein) can also be applied to the wrists, temples and the fontanelle.

Directions are the same as for adults – 4 drops from a prepared treatment bottle either in a little water, milk or fruit juice, and in the case of bottle-fed babies, added to the content of the bottle. When mother is still feeding the baby, she may take the remedies as well, either for herself or for her child, but in taking a remedy for her child's benefit, the effect will not be imparted (through her milk) until about 2 feeds later.

(NOTE: While we consider the Bach Remedies totally safe, it is always recommended that pregnant women consult with their own physician or midwife before taking any therapeutic agent.)

Babies

Many readers ask us how they can prescribe for babies 'for surely they do not suffer from negative states of mind at that age'. Indeed they do, for they have come to earth especially to overcome certain difficulties, and when they can be helped at this early age, their passage through life will be much easier and happier for them.

Ask any mother of a family and she will tell you each of her babies had a personality of its own, and a very definite one. One mother said, "John, my first baby, was a happy little soul, quite content to be left alone at times, sleeping peacefully, gurgling or playing with his toes, smiling at everyone, crying very little and then only for a good reason – he was uncomfortable or wet or not feeling quite so well. Then he would be restless but made little fuss". He was an **Agrimony** baby, "happy and contented" never really worrying others with his troubles. "My second baby, Jane, was quite a different proposition. She wanted attention all the time, she cried a lot and was only comforted if she was picked up and nursed or carried about. She was very fretful if she did not feel well". Jane was a **Chicory** baby, always wanting attention and not happy until she had it.

"Stephen, my third baby, was quite different too. He was a very nervous baby, noise frightened him, loud voices, or any quick movement, and at night he evidently feared the dark so we had to leave the light on for him". His remedy was **Mimulus**, fears of known things. The three babies were treated with their own Remedy – four drops in a teaspoonful of water, four times a day if the baby was breast fed, or four drops of the prepared medicine in the milk bottle. The mother was so grateful, for John and Jane and Stephen grew up into happy healthy children and Stephen, she said, was as brave as a lion.

Then there is the impatient baby with quite a little temper – **Impatiens**. The sleepy drowsy baby who seems to take no notice or interest in anything around him – **Clematis**. It fact very young babies show their greatest difficulty very plainly. Later they will have, no doubt, various temporary moods of negative states of mind, when they can then be treated, but if the type of personality difficulty is treated straight away, the minor ones will easily be conquered.

Children

Children respond wonderfully well on the Remedies, often quicker than adults, because they have no doubting, interfering intellect. Their emotional problems are real enough to them, but fortunately only skin deep and so the correction should not prove too difficult. School environment has proved to be a very traumatic period in the lives of many children . . . examinations and the consequence of failure. The goading, threats, demands on or influence over the more sensitive, junior or physically smaller children by those endowed with stronger personalities and physical strength. The need to be 'accepted' – painful infatuations that secretly create turmoil in the minds of adolescents in addition to so many other experiences that tend to create petty jealousies, envy, pretence, fear, self-consciousness, shyness, timidity, hatred, lack of confidence and so on – they all need due understanding and help. The two extremes – excessive parental control or indifference add but another echelon to the emotional battles a youngster has to endure. Bringing up children to be happy, healthy and sensible human beings is a job which all parents know to be far more complex than appears on the surface. Modern children enjoy a great deal of liberty to develop along their own lines, yet this very liberty, in itself a good thing, can cause a number of problems if it is not wisely directed.

The process of growing up is hard for some and such needy children are perfect subjects for the Bach Remedies and can be helped greatly. It might appear from the foregoing that the sensitive quiet types require preferential treatment due to their apparent 'suffering' – that may be true – but, let us not forget that the bully equally requires help, so that he learns to use his power of mind and body to correct and support, rather than bludgeon and dominate. Let us not forget too the often 'neglected' second or middle child who feels somewhat left out of things when a new arrival comes along. Reaction here can vary from jealousy, resentment, hatred to the feeling of self pity, loneliness, fear that they are no longer loved, etc. etc.

All too often we hear that the modern child is 'whiney' and constantly seeking attention, or that he is disobedient, wilful and thoughtless for others. All children are like this at times, but with a little help the more positive sides of their natures can be helped to mature and these unpleasant moods kept within reasonable limits. Children who are allowed to tyrannise over the household are rarely happy, any more than children who are oppressed.

Mothers sometimes find it difficult to assess the needs of their children and themselves. Perhaps the following will offer some guidance in general.

Agimony: When we want to get away from noise and chatter or have aches and pains to bear.

Impatiens: When time is short and the child is slow. To help us resist the temptation to do everything for the toddler rather than watch its own slow and fumbling efforts to do things for itself. For the infinite patience so necessary always.

Hornbeam: For times when we feel we cannot cope with so many chores and are tired at the very thought.

Cherry Plum: When we feel we would like to 'take it out' on the child because we have reached the end of our endurance. 'The last straw' feeling.

Elm: To help when although we try so hard to be an ideal parent the task seems beyond our mortal scope, and we despair of doing our job well.

As for the child, his needs vary as he grows.

At Birth: **Star of Bethlehem** for the shock which birth must be to a tiny babe, and **Agrimony** to soothe, or simply **Rescue Remedy**.

For very young babies: **Walnut** (for adjustment). **Star of Bethlehem** for many strange sounds which shock the tiny system.

Teething: **Crab Apple** (cleanser), **Impatiens** (impatience and irritability. **Walnut** to help through the time of change.

Temper tantrums: **Impatiens, Holly.**

Timid, shy, 'clinging' children: **Chicory, Mimulus, Larch.**

Fear of Dark, of Mother leaving them alone, of animals, etc: **Mimulus Aspen.**

The bullying child: **Beech, Holly, Vine.**

The child who is never still, wakefulness: **Vervain.**

The drowsy, apathetic child: **Clematis.**

First days at school: **Walnut, Honeysuckle, Mimulus, Olive** (most children become exhausted at this time).

A discriminating and regular use of the Remedies can do so much to give patience, confidence and tolerance to the mother, and help her to rear a happy lively and co-operative child who will meet all new experiences, and the world in general, with confidence and friendliness.

Treatment of
Animals/Plants

I understand that the Remedies can successfully treat animals and plants – is that correct, and what method of diagnosis is used?

Yes indeed. Over the years we have received very excellent reports of animals and plants coming through some very traumatic conditions and situations. Many animals have been given up for 'dead', yet have revived simply through the Rescue Remedy. We do not consider the Rescue to be a panacea for humans, but it certainly can be the main basic remedy in the animal and plant kingdoms. The normal dosage is – for domestic pets, 4 drops in drinking water or milk – some of this can be sprinkled over the animal's food as well. For larger animals – 10 drops per bucket of water – or perhaps 4 drops on a cube of sugar if it is easier to administer. For plants – 10 drops of Rescue Remedy (and 10 drops of Crab Apple if a cleanser is needed) to a 1 gallon watering can.

For diagnosis – try and put yourself in the animal's skin (like a pantomime horse or goose) – consider how you would feel if a certain thing was happening to you. There are signs of course, like the tail between the legs, showing great fear or timidity (Mimulus plus Rescue Remedy). A cat for ever curled up in a chair, and if moved, soon finds another spot to settle down, doesn't like going out (Clematis, Wild Rose). A cow – easily manipulated (Centaury), staring into space and very lethargic (Clematis and Wild Rose). A bull on the other hand is much more aggressive and is a controller of his domain (Vine, Chicory, maybe Cherry Plum for its vile rages).

Nora Weeks used to say that the type remedy for most

cats was Water Violet because of its aloofness, independence and need to go about its own business without interference or involvement in other creatures' affairs (other than mice or birds perhaps!). A dog that growls at anyone nearing their home or master (Chicory, for possessiveness, and Holly for jealousy/suspicion). A plant that has been uprooted accidentally needs Rescue Remedy for shock, but probably Walnut too if it has to be transplanted. Plants can be treated with Rescue Remedy and Crab Apple irrespective on a regular basis – it acts like a natural tonic.

One of our News Letter readers suggested that the combination above of Rescue Remedy and Crab Apple in a watering can virtually cleared black spot from her roses. Rescue Remedy cream can be applied to a damaged tree trunk or branch – this has been known to help 'heal the wound'.

The Bach Centre is always willing to make further suggestions.

The Bach Method
As opposed to alternative
methods used

S IMPLICITY. Dr. Bach's keyword was 'Simplicity'. The final listing of his remedies and their applied mental deviations were presented by him in such a way, that people from all walks of life would be able, without fear or confusion to fully understand his findings, and (perhaps more significantly), be able to diagnose for themselves and friends with absolute impunity.

The true use of the word simplicity has been wrongly misconstrued by some to mean insignificant or infantile. Such phrases as 'higher visions', 'deeper perceptions' are expressed in some circles to convince others that some modern concept or up-dated method of prescribing was long over-due – nothing could be further from the truth. Dr. Bach predicted that this method of healing would be 'the medicine of the future' – a potential that is only now beginning to be fully recognised, so any suggestion that they are outdated or ripe for fresh experimentation is quite misleading. Although there may be many new diseases and also difficult conditions of life – these have happened in every generation – *human nature remains the same*. People still fear and hate, get impatient and resentful, grow hopeless and depressed just as they have done since time immemorial. Our bodily health depends upon the way we face up to the various conditions of life. A negative outlook will affect both the body and the events of our lives, as Job realised when he said "That which I have feared has come upon me". So the 38 Bach Remedies are for all time. *FEAR* of AIDS today is no different to the *FEAR* of DIPHTHERIA in the thirties.

Dr. Bach was indisputably a very highly evolved soul, for whom simplicity meant the purest vision of all, representing the nucleus of all perfection and understanding, unfettered by complexity or dogma.

The following random extracts appeared in early News Letters, written by Nora Weeks and other authorities on the subject. They are included her to confirm that the need to uphold the doctor's original method is paramount in our eyes, not because we are being short-sighted, possessive or narrow minded as some would suggest, but simply to carry out the very wish that Dr. Bach himself expressed – a legacy that is quite sacred and very much incumbent on us as custodians to protect:–

"Before he died, Dr. Bach told us that many would want to add to the number of Remedies, would want to change and complicate the method, but asked us to keep it in its full simplicity, for it was a system of healing which could be used safely by anyone with compassion and understanding. He said also: 'Although this method of treatment is the medicine of the future, and will spread through the world, keep to your simple way of living, which is the true way of living.'

So we still live in the little red brick house standing on the bank at the bend of the lane. We do our own cooking and washing-up and look after the garden. We find that people come from all over the world to see us here and to learn more about Dr. Bach and the Flower Remedies".

Nora Weeks

"We have been told we are too unsophisticated. We are glad about this, for life is simple and can be expressed in words of two syllables – be kind, never hurt others, be happy. We remember also the words of Dr. bach about this work: 'Let not the simplicity of this method deter you from its use, for the further your researches advance the more you will realise the simplicity of all Creation'".

Nora Weeks

"Friends have at different times over the years, expressed concern at the various attempts to destroy the simplicity of Dr. Bach's work, asking what steps if any, we intend to take. We have for a long time been aware of these attempts. Many and varied have been the suggested 'extensions'. Had we accepted these various attempts at distortion, the divine simplicity of the doctor's work would have long ago been utterly destroyed.

All this was foreseen and spoken by Dr. Bach. In October 1936; about a month before he died, he wrote to me:

'This last episode of D.M.W. may be welcomed. It is a proof of the value of our work when material agencies arise to distort it, because attempted distortion is a far greater weapon than attempted destruction. Mankind has asked for freewill, which God granted him; hence mankind must always have a choice. As soon as a teacher has given his work to the world, a contorted version of the same must arise. Such has happened from the humblest like ourselves who have dedicated our services to the good of our fellow-men, even to the Highest of all, the Christ. The contortion must be raised for people to be able to choose between the gold and the dross — *Bach*' "

Victor Bullen

"It has come to our notice that some people are preparing the Bach Remedies by radionic and magno-geometric methods. They say the Remedies are just as effective, but these Remedies must not be called 'Bach Remedies', for no man-made appliances can better Nature's way of preparing the Bach Remedies.

Nature uses the sun, water, the earth and the air together with the *living* wild flowers. The plants grow and gain their food from the soil of their own choice, in the open air. The sun imparts the healing life force from the flowers into the water in the glass bowl, which rests in the actual field where the plants are growing. Then Nature takes it all into her own hands, for, apart from quickly and gently picking the flower heads and putting them on a broad leaf on the collector's hand to prevent their touching the skin before floating them on the water in the glass bowl, all happens without human interference. The flower heads are still fresh and living when the preparation is finished. The water in the bowl is sparkling and full of tiny bubbles — living water, the life force of the flowers.

With the flowers that are boiled in the early part of the year, before the sun has gained its full strength, there is also no human interference apart from the collecting of the flowers. The wild flowers used for the 38 Bach Remedies are those of a very high order. Nature herself grows these flowering plants or trees without the interference of human beings or science. She sees that each grows in the soil that suits it best, that they bloom at the right time and that they are watered by her rain and brought to perfection by the rays of the sun.

Compare this with the preparation by radiesthesia and other apparatus, in a closed room away from the sun and air, no flowers used. There is indeed something vital missing, as you can well understand. People say that modern methods, advanced techniques must take the place of the old simple methods and ideas. But Nature does not change, it is the same whether it is yesterday or today".

Nora Weeks

"Some people find it rather difficult to accept the simple guide lines set down by Dr. Bach. For example, on the matter of dosage it was recently advocated that drops should be in ratio to the size of bottle and dropper used. Such reasoning would be understood if statistics entered into it . . . but that is where the fault lies, in that there is no calculative basis involved.

There is a minimum dosage of 2 drops of any stock remedy to any amount of water, up to 30 mil, when preparing a bottle. When the dosage is taken, it is 4 drops irrespective of the size of the actual treatment bottle that has been prepared.

It is important, please, that people do not make up their own minds concerning what is right and wrong in what they might interpret the Bach Remedies to be – it creates unnecessary confusion that misleads the novice, and those who are easily influenced by persuasion and argument. Let them be guided by the origin of the work that has stood the test for over 55 years. Please refer to our instruction sheet for precise details."

John Ramsell

"Although one would not consider the Bach treatment old enough to have developed some 'old wives' tales', there are certain erroneous statements being included in various 'lectures' and courses of instruction, which cause a certain amount of anxiety amongst those who receive such tuition.

One such tale is that if two Remedy bottles stand side by side without their stoppers one will contaminate the other. Another is that if one should inadvertently touch one's tongue with a dropper, this would in turn affect the stock Remedy. Often we are asked to confirm the fact that a bottle of stock Remedy can be constantly topped up with brandy after use without weakening the power of the Remedy proper. The answer to each of the suggestions is that they are wrong . . . with reference to the last item, the stock bottles will keep indefinitely in their original form, adding brandy will certainly not make them 'everlasting', in fact doing this would be the equivalent of diluting them down into treatment or dosage bottles. We are inclined to think that such teachings are yet again based on alternative ideas. So let us reassure everyone, that each stock Remedy has its own equal strength, that they all marry well with each other on an equal foundation, that they are simple, and natural, and therefore need no extra qualifications other than those that are provided as a guidance from our literature. Pay no heed to those who would impose restrictions by dubious authority, just to make them more complicated".

Nickie Murray

"One of the main virtues of the Bach Remedies is its absolute simplicity which people seem to find so difficult to accept. The flowers supply a need just as readily as hunger can be appeased with food. As Dr. Bach said, 'I want to make it as simple as this: 'I am hungry, I will go and pull a lettuce from the garden for my tea; I am frightened and ill, I will take a dose of Mimulus',' or whatever the condition indicates".

Jane Evans

"It is our privilege and purpose here at Mount Vernon, the Centre of Dr. Bach's method of treatment and the Bach Remedies, to maintain, as he requested before he died in 1936, the simplicity of his work.

Many people throughout the years have suggested that more Remedies should be added, certain changes in their preparation, other more complicated methods of prescribing them. This shows their great interest, but the

Bach Remedies form a system of healing which is unique and complete".

Nora Weeks

"Dr. Bach's work has many followers, hundreds of people throughout the world write asking for help and information, but like all new work it is at times misused and abused.

In view of several recent letters which show that the Remedies have not always been fully understood, it is necessary to warn readers against some of these misunderstandings.

A lady interested in spiritualism wrote to say that she had found many new remedies to add to those of Dr. Bach. She claimed that the plants were found after messages from the spirit world.

Dr. Bach was a physician and surgeon, he was also a bacteriologist and had spent many years in research. He took the greatest care in choosing the Remedies to use only herbs that could have no harmful results if used by non-qualified people. He brought a life-time of experience and research to his work.

However good other herbal remedies may be, they have not been tried and proved by his methods and we cannot allow them to be added to his list.

Attention was also drawn to the case of an osteopath who tried to use the Remedies for injections, with very unfortunate results.

These Remedies have been prepared to be taken by mouth or used as lotions. They were never intended for, and are quite unsuitable for injections.

In these News Letters we have tried to explain the Remedies and their uses in simple straightforward language. We would ask all those interested to beware of treatments offered in the name of Dr. Bach, which do not conform to his methods and standards".

Frances Wheeler

"Looking through the back numbers of the News Letter from 1950, it will be seen that the simplicity of Dr Bach's work has been stressed repeatedly. This has been necessary, not only for the sake of new readers, but because most of us need to be reminded that distortion can easily arise.

Again and again down through the ages the divinely simple message of joy and health given to mankind has been complicated, obscured and distorted out of all recognition.

So once more here is an extract from Dr. Bach's 'Twelve Healers and Other Remedies', printed also in the very first News Letter of March 1950; "There is little more to say for the understanding mind will know all this; and may there be sufficient of those with understanding minds, unhampered by the trend of science, to use these Gifts of God for the relief and the blessing of those around them."

It is indeed remarkable that the above was written by a doctor with much more than a passing knowledge of scientific methods. I quote further from the introduction in *The Twelve Healers*: "No science, no knowledge is necessary, apart from the simple methods described herein, and they who will obtain the greatest benefit from this God-sent Gift will be those who keep it as it is, free from science, free from theories, for everything in nature is simple."

And so it has come to pass, wonderful things have happened and many have been healed by adhering to his simple instructions".

Nora Weeks/Victor Bullen

What is your opinion of various other methods of prescribing the Bach Remedies?

It is of absolute importance that Dr. Bach's concept of prescribing and administering his Remedies be fully understood and accepted by all, as the only method to be taught. We are constantly finding it necessary to explain to people throughout the world, that the proper method of prescribing is as laid down by Dr. Bach himself i.e. by using one's intuition, based on the simple knowledge of each remedy and the states of mind they represent. We know that *experts* in the use of muscle testing, astrological charts and pendulums can obtain positive results through their respective diagnostic methods and subsequent use of the Bach Remedies. We recognise that good results are all that matter in the end, but the problem is that many of these good people become so enthused by their own beliefs and interpretations that they allow any early conviction held of the Bach theory to be overshadowed by their own particular insight. It is then that they fall under the pretext that the remedies are an integral part of *their* work – instead of recognising the Bach

Remedies to be a complete treatment in its own right, granting them, as it does, a very convenient practical therapeutic answer to their diagnostic exercise.

We cannot over-stress the significance and responsibility on all our shoulders in upholding the purity of Dr. Bach's system of prescribing – for once we allow other interpretations (no matter how persuasive they may appear to be) to supersede the long established procedure, the whole foundation of this work will begin to crumble. It was Dr. Bach's dearest wish that his work remain unaltered in its *basic simple form* and we call on all those who respect his name to help ensure the endurance of his trust.

With the advent of so many facsimiles coming forth (especially from America) how can I be certain I am having the genuine Bach Remedies? Some people offer ready-diluted remedies for sale.

First and foremost, ensure that the Bach name and address (the long-hand style of the Bach name is in fact Dr. Bach's own signature – this in itself is very significant) is on the label. We have authorised distributors in many countries (these are listed on our pamphlet), who in turn might need, by law, to add their name to the label in addition to our own. *The preparation of a treatment bottle is only in order when they are being made up for a specific client or patient, we do not agree with such bottles being prepared in advance and sold over the counter as Bach Remedies proper.* A 7.5 ml stock bottle that costs approximately £1.50 should surely not be used as a means of providing a re-sale of 45 bottles containing nothing more than 2 drops of the original stock in alcohol. So ensure that the Bach label is on the bottle as stated above – any other cannot be claimed as a genuine product.

(Note: Bach Flower Remedies and Rescue Remedy are protected titles (trade marked) and therefore cannot be rebottled, other than as a treatment proper.)

Why don't you adopt the convenient method of Remedies in tablet form?

Dr. Bach, as a leading Homoeopathic physician, would have chosen this method had he intended it to be that way. Instead his choice was the liquid form, so that a composite could be made up much more easily by the simple method of putting 2 drops of one's chosen remedies into a 30 ml bottle of water – from which 4 drops would then be taken at least 4 times per day. Consider the difference if one had to purchase the different remedies in tablet form, taking 2 or 3 tablets from *each* bottle throughout the day – it would be quite impractical as you can gather. But in any case the liquid form is more efficient, and allows external application when necessary – which is not possible with tablets. We do recognise the problem that the liquid remedy can create for those who have difficulty in handling things (e.g. the blind, elderly, and those with Parkinson's Disease) or for the occasion when unobtrusiveness is necessary. For such people we can, on request, refer them to an address where Rescue Remedy (only) can be provided in tablet form. (viz. A. Nelson & Co. Ltd., 5 Endeavour Way, Wimbledon, London SW19 9UH.)

A person who prescribed by the pendulum method recently stated that I would need 10 drops of Walnut, 4 drops of Larch and 2 drops of some other remedy . . . is this a new prescribing method that has been found?

No, there is no new method of prescribing – Dr. Bach stipulated 2 drops of any chosen remedy in the one preparation – to use more would do no harm, but would be wasteful. One gains no more, by drinking a whole bottle of any particular Remedy in stock concentrate form, than in having 2 drops of that same remedy in a glass of water – the taking of more drops will have NO ENHANCED EFFECT WHATSOEVER. Any variation as suggested in the question is entirely wrong and misleading.

We have already mentioned in answer to a question on page 106 that good results *have* been forthcoming from those who have the innate ability to use the pendulum properly, but we are coming across many novices who claim that they need to turn to this medium to gain ratification when they are uncertain about their own judgment or intuition in prescribing. This conjours up rather an important question as to which remedy would they choose, if the pendulum delivered a different answer to their original choice? Also – when another person's advice is sought, to determine a choice of remedy, and the friend's 'pendulum reading' decrees an entirely different remedy (as is quite often the case we have been told) . . . what then?! We would like beginners to learn the Bach method thoroughly – so that the choice of remedies becomes automatic, then there would be no doubt in their ability to prescribe properly. So much better surely than getting themselves bogged down by so many confusing suggestions, causing unnecessary mistakes, that can be of little use to their own aspirations, and most certainly, be of little solace to those relying on them for help.

(A point of interest – the afore-mentioned novices who need to seek confirmation because they lack confidence in their own judgment, could do with a good dose of CERATO!)

Are there more Remedies to be found?

In relation to the Bach Flower Remedies the answer is NO (see Introduction page 12).

How therefore do foreign and other flower essences relate to Dr. Bach's findings?

We have never made a secret of the origin or methodology involved in Dr. Bach's discoveries. In fact a book was written by Nora Weeks and Victor Bullen in 1964, which openly described the various plants used and how they were made. The intention of this book was to provide the means of finding and making the remedies for those, in this country, who would wish to make some remedies for their own use. Nora withdrew this book before she died because she was greatly concerned that it was being exploited commercially. Dr. Bach used two methods of preparing his remedies – the plants that mature in the early part of the year when there is little sunshine (mainly the flowers and twigs of the trees and bushes) are prepared by the 'boiling method', whereas the flowers blooming during the late spring and in the summer when the sun is at the height of its power are prepared by the 'Sun method', with exceptions that are prepared by boiling. The 'Sun method' was Dr. Bach's own unique creation. After discovering the healing quality of a particular flower, he required to find a means of harnessing this healing quality. He realized it was entirely out of the question to offer the flowers themselves, but then, due to the development of his sensitivity in that he was able to place the petal of a flower on his tongue or lay it on the palm of his hand and take on the properties of that plant, he found that a dew drop, having basked on a flower for a little while in the sunshine, actually contained the same quality as the plant itself – in other words, the sun had extracted into the sparkling dew drop its healing quality. Dr. Bach then actually began to gather these drops of dew into bottles, because he now had a means of administering the flower remedy, but he soon realized that such a method was far too involved and time consuming, so a more practical system had to be devised. It was then that he envisaged in his mind the picture of a 'larger dew drop' in the form of a clear glass bowl, filled with pure spring water, with the surface covered by the flower heads – this to stand in the warm sunshine for 3 hours in a position as near as possible to the mother plant. As with the dew drop, the spring water became impregnated with the healing properties of the plant . . . and so the system of preparation was born.

Recently this method of preparation has been adopted to convert long established herbal remedies proper (that would normally be used in root or dried form to cure a wide spectrum of physical diseases and general conditions, which are also credited to have some effect on the patient's mental state) into liquid form (over 500 of these have been prepared in recent years). It would be incorrect to call these 'flower essences' – what they truly are, are liquid herbal essences, which have no direct association to Dr. Bach's findings whatsoever. There are many books on the subject of Herbalism proper, and of course, it is fully recognized by ourselves that the hundreds of herbs are, in their own right, fully established as healing remedies, and have been for centuries. Take Borage Offici-analis for example, which affords a well known range of medicinal uses ranging from reducing fevers and helping pulmonary complaints, to acting as a poultice for inflammatory swelling. These qualities are fully described in "A Modern Herbal" volume I. Cape, London, which also attributes Borage to having the following effect on the emotions: (note the ancient script form) – "The leaves and floures of Borage put into wine make men and women glad and merry and drive away all sadnesse, dul-nesse and melancholy, as Diosorides and Pliney affirme". **It must be stressed that Dr. Bach by-passed all such references – he did not resort to discovering what had already been written by earlier scribes.** It was pure coinci-dence if any of Dr. Bach's findings happened also to be used in Herbalism – one example of this would be Ver-vain, and it soon becomes obvious that the doctor's find-ings were entirely apart from the herbal descriptions and correlations. Dr. Bach endured 6 years of privation as well as mental and physical suffering in discovering and developing his 38 specific remedies – specific in that Gorse for example, deals with the state of hopelessness – it has no other function. This fact applies to each and every one of his choice of flowers, the related states of mind for each being absolutely original and very special – simple to understand and simple to use.

The suggestion that Dr. Bach's findings are now outdated and that new offerings carry on where he left off is quite wrong – for despite changing conditions of life and modern influences, human nature remains the same. People all over the world still fear and hate, get impatient and resentful, grow hopeless and depressed, lose confidence or become self-conscious just as they have done since time immemorial – so the Bach Flower Remedies are for all time and for the benefit of all people irrespective of their nationality. Nora Weeks, who worked throughout with the doctor, became his rightful heir and as such, she, and she alone, held the privileged right to choose in turn her successors. Those of us who were appointed by her carry on their hereditary duties accordingly, having in turn been empowered to determine the future curators of the Bach Centre and the work when it befalls them to make the choice.

Dr. Bach's selection of plants was not based on genus/species alone – his great sensitivity narrowed his choice of some plants to a very fine point of selectivity. For example, the Impatiens flower offers two shades of colouring, but Dr. Bach determined that the healing quality of this plant was obtained only from the one particular colour of petal. Apart from the exceptions, Vine, Olive, Cerato and course Rock Water (this being the odd one in that it is of a natural healing spring water), the Bach Flower Remedies are indigenous to this country. We were recently in touch with the Royal Botanic Gardens in Kew (internationally renowned authority) and they volunteered the following information concerning overseas plants – "It might be inadvisable to introduce plants from other areas, and possibly of overseas origin, without first checking natural genetic variability of the species concerned". This statement reiterates what has always been stated over the years – Nora Weeks wrote in her very last News Letter (written before her passing in Jan. 1978) the following declaration: "We wish to impress upon those in England who would attempt to prepare their own essences of the Bach Flowers, that they take infinite care to select the right flowers, otherwise they will be disappointed with the results. We also ask those living abroad not to prepare the essences, even if the flowers have the same Latin names, for, due to the difference in soil and climate they will not have the desired effect".

It has been suggested that one should prepare oneself through meditation prior to making Mother Tinctures – how is your ritual carried out?

Most of us have, over the years, taken the part of the 'Good Samaritan', giving or helping those in need, whether it be to the benefit of our own families, or to little children or even outsiders . . . it is the great pleasure of giving, seeing the warmth of gratitude in an elderly person's face or the twinkle of sheer excitement in the eye of a child at Christmas time, that offers the giver a sense of joy and pleasure that has a special "feel" about it.

Nora Weeks and Victor Bullen and likewise ourselves have always recognized Nature as the great provider, smiling on us year in year out generously offering us its precious bounty – and we become, as with the elderly person or child, so very appreciative of God's wonderful gifts.

We cannot understand therefore why the suggestion should be made, that before making the Remedies, we should "attune or prepare ourselves in some meditative sense" . . . as in the way of some Mystic perhaps? Surely, there is no need to work oneself up into a preparatory state before giving thanks or offering a prayer to one's Maker? – this can be carried out by sincere thought alone, as one can sense a closeness to a distant relative by simply re-calling to mind a happy recollection, or vision of that person's face. It is similar to that profound love or affinity that we can sense between ourselves and others, when there is no uneasiness or strain present to mar the occasion, or when one feels at home and at ease, even in the presence of a complete stranger . . . these are the *natural qualities* that help to create an immediate rapport or bond between souls, in all forms of Creation. Our association with plant life is born of this (common to us all) innate quality.

So – when everything is right – the climate, the plant itself at its zenith – we set forth. The uplift of a sunny day, and our venturing into the countryside to perform our heritable task of making the Mother Tinctures, auto-matically attunes us to the 'right state of mind'. Nothing is taken for granted, for we are fully aware that without these precious gifts that we have been privileged to pro-cure, there would be no Bach Remedies. In the realization of all this, it is only necessary, that we do not forget to say "Thank you".

———————

Due to world-wide development of hundreds of 'flower essences' these last number of years, all being made through Dr. Bach's Sun Method of preparation and thereby associated with his name, it became necessary for us to establish legal protection to ensure the purity, originality and perhaps more so to safeguard the long established good name of Dr. Bach's findings. All Dr. Bach's choice of remedies are harmless and proved themselves to be so for over 55 years, with no complaint of any consequence ever being levelled against them. Many medicinal plants require to be prepared under expert guidance and experience, as under Herbalism proper, homoeopathy or Allopathy, but become questionable if prepared by any other 'uncontrolled' method – e.g. Belladonna, Euphorbia, Ragwort, Jonquils. The latter for instance is referred to in 'A Modern Herbal' (M. Grieve), which states, ". . . the flowers are considered slightly poisonous and have been known to have produced dangerous effects upon children" – yet it is prepared in one particular country – 'For demanding children sensitive to family tensions.'

People with any regard for Dr. Bach would fully realize the difficult dilemma that is created when his name becomes associated with this sort of activity. In the event of someone suffering illness or something more serious as a result of taking such remedies, the method of preparation would undoubtedly come under scrutiny, and this would inevitably, in the eyes of the authorities lead to a question mark of doubt being levelled, most unfairly and unwarranted at the Bach Flower Remedies themselves!

(See Dr. Bach's letter to Victor Bullen on page 99).

We trust that this booklet has helped to bring you up to date on many issues and that you now feel able to answer some questions with a feeling of 'authority'. If any reader has further questions, that often crop up, then please let us have them and they will be considered for future issues.

For the benefit of those overseas the following are our official foreign distributors:

USA: Ellon (Bach U.S.A.) Inc., P.O. Box 320, Woodmere, N.Y., 11598 U.S.A. (Tel: 516 593 2206).

Canada: Bach (Canada), P.O. Box 2465, Peterborough, Ontario, Canada K9J 7Y8. (Tel: (705) 749–1894).

Germany/Austria: Dr. Bach-Blüten-Essenzen-Handelsges. mbH (Bach Centre German Office, M. Scheffer), Eppendorfer Landstraße 32., D-2000 Hamburg 20. (Tel: 040-46 10 41).

Switzerland: Dr. Bach-Blüten AG (Bach Centre Swiss Office), Alte Landstraße 57, CH-8700 Küsnacht. (Tel: 01-911 09 11)

Australia: Martin & Pleasance Pty. Ltd., P.O. Box 2054, Richmond, Vic. 3121, Australia. (Tel: 427 7422).

Holland/Benelux: Holland Pharma, Postbus 37, 7240 AA Lochem, Holland. (Tel: 05730-2884)

Belgium: Aquila PVBA. Ch de Beriotstraat 2, B-3000 Leuven, Belgium. (Tel. 16 229501).

Denmark: Camette, Lillebaeltsvej 47, 6715 Esbjerg, Denmark. (Tel 05-1833556).

Italy: Guna, via Staro 10, 20134 Milano, Italy. (Tel. 039 2 2155107).

Die Leo, via Kennedy, 13-40069 Zola Predosa (BO). Italy. (Tel. 051/75.46.10).

France: M. Jean Revillon, 'La Jonquille', 7 Route de Fournes, Escobecques, 59320 Haubourdin, France. (Tel. 20.07.63.97).

M.F. Deporte, Lasserre s.a., BP. 4, La Sableyre-Illats, 33 720 Podensac, France. (Tel. 56.62.57.00).

New Zealand: Weleda (N.Z.) Ltd., Box 132, Havelock North, Hawke's Bay, New Zealand. (Tel. (070) 777 394).

ALL ORDERS FOR REMEDIES AND BOOKS, AND ALL MATTERS CONCERNING DISTRIBUTION, MARKETING AND GENERAL SALES CONTACT: Bach Flower Remedies, Unit 6, Suffolk Way, Drayton, Abingdon, Oxon. OX14 5JX (Tel. 0235 550086: Fax: 523973) All information concerning other foreign distributors not listed above can be obtained from this source.

ADVICE, ORDERS FOR THE BACH CENTRE'S NEWSLETTERS, TREATMENTS, CONSULTATIONS AND VISITATIONS (by prior appointment), APPLICATION FOR SEMINARS AND COURSES and etc. CONTACT: The Bach Centre, Mount Vernon, Sotwell, Wallingford, Oxon. OX10 OPZ. (Tel. 0491 34678: Fax: 25022. The Centre is open normally for brief visits and small purchases between 10 a.m. and 3 p.m. Mon. to Fri. inclusive – closed Bank Holidays and weekends).

We list below the various Bach books that are already translated and sold in foreign countries – these are not available through the Bach Centre (UK).

USA/CANADA

'The Medical Discoveries of Edward Bach'; 'The Handbook of the BFR'; 'The Bach Flower Remedies' (*one book combining Heal Thyself. Twelve Healers and Repertory*). *Publisher*: Keats Publishing Inc., 212 Elm St., New Canaan, Connecticut, USA. (Note: other books in English are stocked by our U.S. Distributor).

FRANCE

'La Guerison par les Fleurs' (*as USA – 3 booklets in one*).
'Handbook of the Bach Flower Remedies.'
Publisher: Le Courrier du Livre, 21 rue de Seine, Paris 6e, France.

GERMANY

'Blumen die Unsere Seele Heilen' (*3 booklets in one plus coloured illustrations*).
'The Medical Discoveries of Edward Bach'.
Publisher: H. Hugendubel, Nymphenburger Str. 25– 27, 8000 Munchen, W. Germany.
'Handbook of the Bach Flower Remedies'.
Publisher: Aquamarin Verlag, Voglherd 1, D-8018 Grafing, Germany,
(Note: Separate edition availabe is 'Erfahrungen mit der Bach Blutentherapie' and 'Bach Blutentherapie' by M. Scheffer – published by Hugendubel). (Future publications planned – 'Questions and Answers/

Step by Step'; 'Orig. Writings of Dr. Bach';
'Illustrations and Preparations'.

HOLLAND

'Medische Ontdekkingen van Edward Bach' *publisher:*
De Ster – Ginnenkenweg 124, 4818 Breda,
Holland.

'Handboek voor de Bloesemtherapie' *publisher:*
Ankh-Hermes, Smyrn str, 5, Deventer, Holland.

'Genezing door Bloemen' (*3 in one*) *publisher:* De
Driehoek, Keizersgracht, 756, Amsterdam,
Holland.

'Over de Bach Bloemenremedies' *published by:* La
Riviere & Voorhoeve, Gildestr. 5, 8263 Kampen,
Holland.

ITALY

'Guarire con I Fliori' (*2 booklets in one*).
Publisher: IPSA Editore snc, Via Crispi 50–52, 90145
Palermo, Italy.

SPAIN

'La Curacion por las Flores' (*3 booklets in one*).
Publisher: EDAF, Ediciones – distribuciones, S.A. Jorge
Juan, 30. Madrid.

FINLAND

'Paranna Itsesi' (Heal Thyself)
Publisher: Lisi Suokkonen, Uudenmaankatu, 13b,
00120, Helsinki.

ISRAEL

'Handbook of the Bach Flower Remedies'
Publisher: Or'Am Publishing House, 2 Dov Friedman
Street, P.O. Box 22096, Tel Aviv.

GREECE

'Heal Thyself & Twelve Healers' combined in Greek.
Publisher: Theophanes D. Boukas, 73 Skoofa St., 10 6
  80 Athens.
'Handbook of the Bach Flower Remedies'.
Publisher: Kastaniotis Editions, 3 Zoodochou Pigia
  Str., Athens 142.

DENMARK

Please contact our distributor – CAMETTE (address
  on page 117).

Index

Questions under Practical use of the Remedies: